Date Due

JUL 0 8 96			
JUN 19 2000			
DEC 0 1 2005			

BRODART, CO.   Cat. No. 23-233-003   Printed in U.S.A.

Practical Interventional Uroradiology

PRACTICAL

Interventional Uroradiology

edited by

DAVID RICKARDS FRCR, FFRDSA
Consultant Radiologist, The Middlesex Hospital, London

SIMON JONES MRCP, FRCR
Consultant Radiologist, Poole and the Royal Bournemouth Hospital NHS Trusts

KEN R THOMSON FRACR, FRCR
Department of Radiology, The Royal Melbourne Hospital, Melbourne

MATTHEW D RIFKIN MD
Professor and Chairman, Department of Radiology, Albany Medical College, Albany, New York

Edward Arnold
A division of Hodder & Stoughton
LONDON BOSTON MELBOURNE AUCKLAND

First published in Great Britain 1993

Distributed in the Americas by Little, Brown and Company,
34 Beacon Street, Boston, MA 02108

British Library Cataloguing in Publication Data
Rickards, David
    Practical Interventional Uroradiology
    I. Title
    616.6

    ISBN 0-340-55258-X

Whilst the advice and information in this book is believed to be true
and accurate at the date of going to press, neither the author nor the
publisher can accept any legal responsibility or liability for any errors
or omissions that may be made. In particular (but without limiting
the generality of the preceding disclaimer) every effort has been
made to check drug dosages; however, it is still possible that errors
have been missed. Furthermore, dosage schedules are constantly
being revised and new side effects recognised. For these reasons the
reader is strongly urged to consult the drug companies' printed
instructions before administering any of the drugs recommended in
this book.

Photoset in Linotron 202 Bembo by
Rowland Phototypesetting Limited, Bury St Edmunds, Suffolk.
Printed and bound in Great Britain for Edward Arnold, a division of
Hodder and Stoughton Limited, Mill Road, Dunton Green,
Sevenoaks, Kent TN13 2YA by Butler and Tanner Limited,
Frome, Somerset.

Preface

There is no shortage of books on interventional radiology, many of them dedicated to the urinary tract. In agreeing to edit another one, albeit part of an informal series of books on interventional subjects, we had to be sure that there was a place for our format and that the hard work which would be involved would be worth it. To this end, we have assembled a group of contributors, some world renowned, others well known in their own countries and some who are at the start of their careers who have clearly developed an expertise in a specific field of uroradiological investigation and diagnosis that warranted their inclusion. In a discipline that demands close cooperation between specialties, this is reflected in our author list who are radiologists and urologists from the UK, USA and Australia.

What we asked of our contributors was how and why they do interventional procedures. It is therefore a personal portrayal of each author's extensive experience, not an exhaustive review of the literature and a detailing of minutiae with hundreds of unread computer-generated references listed! Some have detailed the equipment they prefer and how they get out of common complications that relentlessly dog interventional diagnostic and therapeutic procedures. The book includes the use of lasers in the urinary tract, a field that is developing rapidly and is set to enhance the use of minimally invasive techniques further. Although not strictly interventional, methods of diagnosis that involve physiological measurements have been included as has a chapter on the commonly seen endoprostheses that are inserted into the urinary tract.

Dr David Rickards   Professor Matt Rifkin
Dr Simon Jones   Dr Ken Thomson
1993

Contents

Contributors

Archie Alexander, MD,
Department of Radiology, Thomas Jefferson University Hospital, Philadelphia

Joseph Bonn, MD,
Department of Radiology, Thomas Jefferson University Hospital, Philadelphia

Timothy J. Christmas, MD, FRCS(Urol.),
Department of Urology, Charing Cross Hospital, London

Rick I. Feld, MD,
Department of Radiology, Thomas Jefferson University Hospital, Philadelphia

Simon J. Hampson, MChir, FRCS(Urol.),
Department of Urology, The Middlesex Hospital, London

Simon A. V. Holmes, FRCS(Ed),
Department of Urology, St Bartholomew's Hospital, London

Simon Jones, MRCP, FRCR,
Departments of Radiology, Poole and Royal Bournemouth Hospital NHS Trusts

Michael J. Kellett, FRCR,
Department of Radiology, St Peter's Hospital, London

Roger S. Kirby, MA, MD, FRCS(Urol.),
Department of Urology, St Bartholomew's Hospital, London

William R. Lees, FRCR,
Department of Radiology, The Middlesex Hospital, London

Euan Milroy, FRCS,
Department of Urology, The Middlesex Hospital, London

Jeremy Noble, FRCS,
Department of Urology, Battle Hospital, Reading

David Rickards, FRCR, FFRDSA,
Department of Radiology, The Middlesex Hospital, London

Matthew D. Rifkin, MD,
Department of Radiology, Albany Medical College, Albany, New York

Ken R. Thomson, FRACR, FRCR,
Department of Radiology, The Royal Melbourne Hospital, Melbourne

Neale A. Walters, FRACR,
Department of Radiology, The Royal Melbourne Hospital, Melbourne

Graham Watson, MD, FRCS(Urol.),
Department of Urology, St Peter's Hospital and The Whittington Hospital, London

CHAPTER 1

The anatomy of the urinary tract

Jeremy Noble and David Rickards

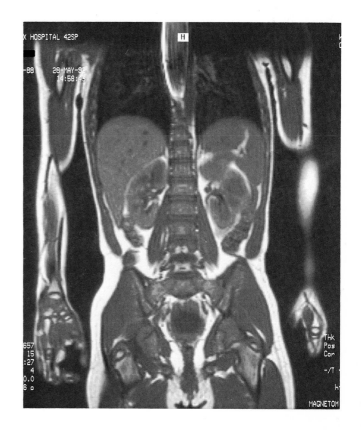

INTRODUCTION

For a surgeon operating on the urinary tract, a complete understanding of the anatomy of the region and a knowledge of the normal variants that occur are all pre-requisites before a procedure. With the advance of radiologically guided interventional techniques, intervention in the urinary tract has become a multidisciplinary procedure involving both urologists and radiologists. Where intervention involves 'closed' techniques and important anatomical structures are not directly visible, a detailed knowledge of urinary tract anatomy is even more relevant.

THE KIDNEYS

General anatomy

The kidneys lie on the posterior abdominal wall on either side of the vertebral column and have a characteristic shape comprising upper and lower poles, a gently convex lateral border and an indented medial border. The hilum of the kidney is situated at the medial border along with the renal pelvis (Fig. 1.1). Each kidney is about 11 cm long, 6 cm wide and 3 cm thick, and in the adult it weighs 135–150 g. The left kidney is often slightly longer and thinner than the right one. The exact position of each kidney is variable being determined by the topography of the muscles of the posterior abdominal wall, but follows a basic general pattern. They lie, within the retroperitoneum, in an oblique position such that the upper pole is nearer to the midline than the lower pole. The majority of kidneys rest between the 1st and 3rd lumbar vertebrae, the right slightly lower due to the liver superiorly. The plane of the renal pelvis is at about 45° to the sagittal plane and the normal lumbar lordosis results in the lower poles lying on a more anterior plane to the superior poles.

The perirenal tissues and retroperitoneum

The kidneys are invested with a continuous covering of fibrous tissue, the renal capsule. This capsule exerts a resting tension upon the underlying renal tissue such that if it is punctured or cut then renal tissue herniates through the capsule. Surrounding the kidneys and their capsules is perirenal fat (Fig.

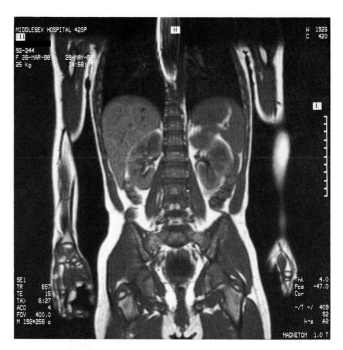

Fig. 1.1 Coronal magnetic resonance scan showing the normally sited kidneys.
They rest on the iliopsoas muscle with the hilum at the level of L1–2. The lower poles are lateral and anterior to the upper poles. Lower pole punctures necessitate the guidewire to pass posteriorly towards the renal pelvis.

1.2). This fat is enclosed by a condensation of transversalis fascia known as the renal fascia, which is itself surrounded by pararenal fat. The renal fascia possesses anterior and posterior layers which subdivide the retroperitoneal tissues on each side of the midline into three potential spaces: the posterior, intermediate and anterior pararenal spaces. The posterior space can be traced anterolaterally, where it is continuous with the space between transversalis fascia and the peritoneum, and only contains fat. The intermediate space, known as the perirenal space, contains the kidney, suprarenal gland and perirenal fat. The anterior space extends across the midline and merges with that of the other side in front of the aorta. Being bounded by the anterior renal fascia and by the parietal peritoneum it contains the retroperitoneal structures of the abdomen, namely the ascending and descending colon, the duodenal loop and the pancreas. Superiorly the two layers of renal fascia merge to the suprarenal gland and blend with the diaphragmatic fascia. Inferiorly they become thin and ill-defined and pass towards the iliac fossa in the shape of a cone whose apex is directed inferiorly. The two layers fuse laterally to form the lateroconal fascia which fuses with the peritoneum of the paracolic gutter having passed posteriorly to the ascending or descending colon. Thus the two layers of the

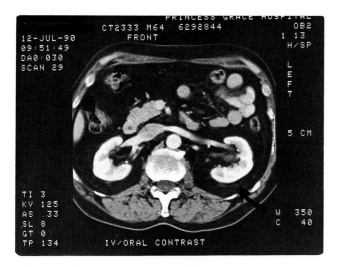

Fig. 1.2 Enhanced transverse axial computed tomographic scan at the level of the renal hila. Both renal veins are readily identified draining into the inferior vena cava. The perinephric fascia posterior to the left kidney can also be seen (arrow).

renal fascia form a closed compartment. The clinical significance of this is that exudate, blood or pus etc. originating from the kidney tends not to cross the midline but usually track down inferiorly to the iliac fossa.

The relations of the kidney

The posterior relations of the right and left kidneys are similar on both sides and are thus considered together. The diaphragm separates the upper pole from the costodiaphragmatic recess of the pleura and the 11th and 12th ribs. Below this the kidneys lie on psoas muscle, quadratus lumborum and transversus abdominis from the medial to lateral positions. Quadratus lumborum is crossed by the subcostal nerve and vessels and the iliohypogastric and ilioinguinal nerves.

Anteriorly the upper pole of the right kidney is capped by the suprarenal gland. The hilum is related to the descending part of the duodenum and the lower pole to the hepatic flexure laterally and duodenal cap medially. The remainder of the anterior surface of the right kidney is related to the visceral surface of the liver. The suprarenal gland lies at the superomedial border of the left kidney and adjacent to this lies the stomach and then the spleen. The tail of the pancreas and splenic vessels crosses the hilum of the left kidney. Inferiorly the lower pole is related to the jejunum medially and splenic flexure laterally.

At the hilum of the kidney the renal vein, renal artery and renal pelvis lie in that order passing posteriorly. A thorough knowledge of the subdivisions of the renal artery is essential with any closed or open intervention and is discussed further. The renal pelvis passes through the hilum into a narrow space, the renal sinus, and is formed by two, or occasionally three, large major calyces. These in turn are formed by three of four minor calyces. Each minor calyx is a trumpet-shaped structure which surrounds either a single papilla or, more rarely, groups of two or three papillae. The renal sinus contains, in addition to the proximal part of the urinary tract, several arteries and veins along with adipose tissue which is continuous with the perirenal fat.

Blood supply of the kidneys

The renal arteries arise from the aorta, the right usually a little lower than the left, and pass towards the renal hilum between the renal vein anteriorly and the renal pelvis posteriorly. The arteries then bifurcate into anterior and posterior branches (Fig. 1.3). From the anterior branch apical, upper anterior, middle anterior and inferior anterior branches appear. These are segmental arteries each supplying a distinct region of the renal parenchyma. The apical branch supplies the upper pole whilst the upper and middle branches supply the anterior surface of the kidney almost equally. The upper vessel usually crosses anterior to the upper pole infundibulum and lies just beneath the mucosa. Evidently, care must be taken in passing rigid endoscopes into this region.

The lower pole segmental artery is the most important vessel to the interventional radiologist as most percutaneous approaches will pass through the parenchyma that this artery supplies, i.e. the anterior and posterior inferior surfaces of the lower pole. The posterior segment of the lower segmental artery curves around the lower pole infundibulum and can be seen pulsating beneath the mucosa at endoscopy.

The posterior artery passes posteriorly to the renal pelvis supplying the parenchyma between the apical and lower segments.

Variations on this pattern are very common and supernumerary renal arteries are present in approximately 20% of individuals.

The veins of the kidney freely intercommunicate with each other (Fig. 1.4). There is no major renal branch to correspond to the posterior renal artery. The posterior veins pass anteriorly to join the renal vein at the necks of the calyces producing a rich venous plexus. If traumatized this plexus will bleed

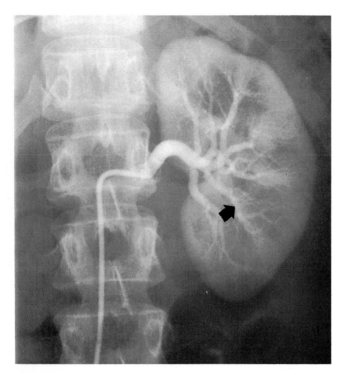

Fig. 1.3 Normal renal angiogram of the left kidney. A lower pole vessel (arrow) can usually be seen at endoscopy pulsating beneath the urothelium covering the lower pole infundibulum. Direct puncture of this area is likely to lead to unnecessary haemorrhage. The vessel medial to this is a branch of the posterior renal artery that supplies the interpolar region of the posterior aspect of the kidney.

but this can usually be stopped by tamponade with a large nephrostomy tube.

THE PELVIURETERIC JUNCTION AND URETER

General anatomy

The ureters are narrow, muscular tubes conveying urine from the kidneys to the bladder at intermittent peristaltic pressures between 20 and 60 cm H_2O and may be as long as 30 cm in the adult male. The upper part of the ureter lies within the retroperitoneum and follows a similar course in the male and the female. The pelvic ureter has a different course in each sex.

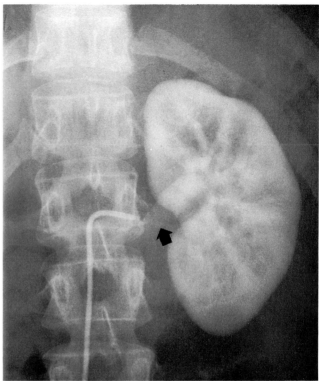

Fig. 1.4 Venous phase of a renal angiogram. Unlike the intrarenal arteries, the veins freely intercommunicate and drain into the renal vein (arrow).

Relations of the ureters

ABDOMINAL URETER

The right ureter passes down towards the pelvis lying on the psoas muscle and crosses the genitofemoral nerve. Anteriorly it is crossed by the descending part of the duodenum, the right colic, middle colic and gonadal vessels and the root of the mesentery (Fig. 1.5). The left ureter has similar posterior relations but is crossed anteriorly by the left colic and gonadal vessels, the root of the sigmoid mesocolon. Both ureters are adherent to the peritoneum of the posterior abdominal wall. Supernumerary renal arteries may cross the ureter either anteriorly or posteriorly resulting in structural and occasionally functional ureteric narrowing.

PELVIC URETER

In the male the ureter crosses the common iliac vessels in front of the sacroiliac joint and then descends on the pelvic side wall to the level of the ischial spine. It then turns medially and forwards around the upper border of the levator ani. The ductus deferens crosses the ureter superiorly from

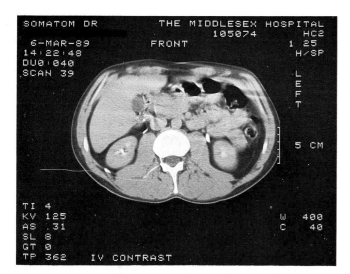

Fig. 1.5 Contrast-enhanced transverse axial computed tomographic scan showing the contrast filled ureters and their close relationship to the iliopsoas muscle.

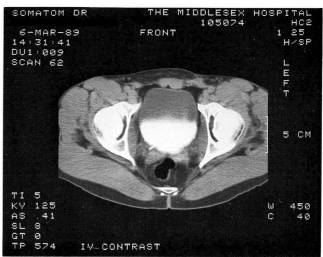

Fig. 1.6 Contrast-enhanced transverse axial computed tomographic scan at a level just superior to the vesicoureteric junction. The contrast filled right ureter can be seen in the angle formed between the right seminal vesicle and the posterior aspect of the bladder.

lateral to medial adjacent to the ischial spine. Just prior to its passage through the bladder wall the ureter is closely related to the tip of the seminal vesicle on its medial side (Fig. 1.6).

In the female the ureter follows a similar route but as it turns medially from the ischial spine it passes under the root of the broad ligament. Here it is often closely related to the ovary in nulliparous women. It is crossed superiorly by the uterine artery and lies in close proximity to the lateral fornix of the vagina. It is here that the ureter is in most danger of damage during a hysterectomy and, it is said, the only place where a ureteric stone may be clinically palpated.

Blood supply of the ureters

The upper third of the ureter is supplied principally from branches arising from the renal artery supplemented by contributions from the gonadal and colic vessels. The middle third supply is extremely variable with branches directly from the aorta and gonadal and iliac vessels. In a small proportion of individuals blood may only be received from peritoneal vessels. This is of considerable clinical relevance as overjudicious mobilization or endoscopic trauma to the ureter may render a portion ischaemic with the risk of subsequent stricture formation. The pelvic ureter receives blood from the vesical, uterine and middle rectal arteries.

Radiological considerations

Despite considerable variation between individuals the bony landmarks of the course of the ureter may be summarized as follows. The region loosely referred to as the pelviureteric junction by clinicians lies just laterally to the tip of the transverse process of the 2nd lumbar vertebra. From here the ureters course down towards the pelvis crossing the tips of the transverse processes of the lumbar vertebrae and then pass laterally over the sacroiliac joints. From here they pass to the level of the ischial spines to pass into the bladder. The site of the ureteric orifices lies over the lateral aspects of the sacrococcygeal joint 3 cm apart. The ureter at the vesicoureteric junction is less distensible than other parts along its course and is a common site for calculi to lodge. Other areas which are said to be narrow are at the pelviureteric junction and the pelvic brim. Narrowings also occur at the site of vessels crossing the ureter, for example, gonadal or supernumerary renal vessels.

THE URINARY BLADDER

General anatomy

The urinary bladder is a reservoir which is designed to store urine at low intravesical pressures. It is a hollow muscular organ lying in the anterior part of the pelvis. The shape of the bladder is highly variable but when empty can be considered as a tetrahedron presenting an apex behind the pubic symphysis, a base and a superior and two inferolateral surfaces. The apex is directed upwards and forwards and is connected to the median umbilical ligament, a remnant of the urachus. This fibrous cord ascends in the extraperitoneal tissues of the anterior abdominal wall as far as the umbilicus. As the bladder fills it becomes ovoid and bulges up from beneath the symphysis pubis behind the anterior abdominal wall. This makes it readily accessible to the clinician for examination, ultrasound and the insertion of suprapubic drainage catheters.

The ureters enter the posterolateral angles of the bladder base and the urethra leaves inferiorly from the bladder neck. The bladder is covered by peritoneum on its superior surface, or fundus, passing posteriorly onto the uterus in the female and the rectum in the male. These folds of peritoneum form the uterovesical and rectovesical pouches, respectively.

The urinary bladder is surrounded by pelvic fascia which becomes thickened to form the ligaments of the bladder, namely, the pubovesical/puboprostatic, lateral and posterior ligaments. In the male the prostate also lends considerable support to the bladder whereas the female bladder tends to be more mobile.

Relations of the urinary bladder

These are obviously different in each sex and are therefore considered separately.

THE MALE

Several nerves and vessels are related to the bladder as it approaches the pelvic side wall. These include the obturator nerve and vessels and the superior vesical artery which continues anteriorly as the obliterated umbilical artery. The seminal vesicle and the ampulla of the ductus deferens are applied to the inferolateral surface of the bladder. When the bladder and/or rectum is full the ampulla of the rectum becomes closely related to the posterior surface of the bladder separated by only the peritoneal layers of the rectovesical pouch. When empty, small bowel often fills the rectovesical pouch separating the bladder from the rectum.

Anteriorly, between the pubic bones and the bladder, lies the retropubic space containing adipose tissue and the pubovesical and puboprostatic ligaments. It is into this space that the bladder expands as

it fills displacing the peritoneum from the anterior abdominal wall. Thus the distended bladder is in direct contact with the anterior abdominal wall and can be approached with a suprapubic catheter introducer without entering the peritoneal cavity.

THE FEMALE

The relations of the female bladder differ posteriorly where it is closely related to the cervix of the uterus and the vagina. Inferiorly the bladder lies in a lower position in the female than in the male and is in close contact with the muscles of the pelvic floor and the perineum.

The blood supply of the urinary bladder

The urinary bladder receives its blood supply from branches of the internal iliac artery. The large superior vesical arteries run along the lateral wall of the pelvis, dividing into two or more terminal branches before reaching the bladder. The smaller inferior vesical arteries supply the base of the bladder along with small direct branches from the internal iliac arteries. The blood drains to a vesical venous plexus lying close to the bladder neck with free communication with the prostatic or vaginal plexuses of veins. These all drain to the internal iliac veins although extensive interconnections exist with plexuses draining the other pelvic organs.

THE MALE URETHRA

General anatomy

The male urethra is an S-shaped tube about 20 cm long conveying urine from the bladder neck to urethral meatus through the prostate gland, deep perineal pouch and the corpus spongiosum. It can be considered to consist of four parts:

1 Preprostatic portion
2 Prostatic urethra
3 Subprostatic urethra
4 Penile urethra

The preprostatic portion of the urethra extends for approximately 1.5 cm from the bladder neck to the base of the prostate gland. The prostatic urethra is

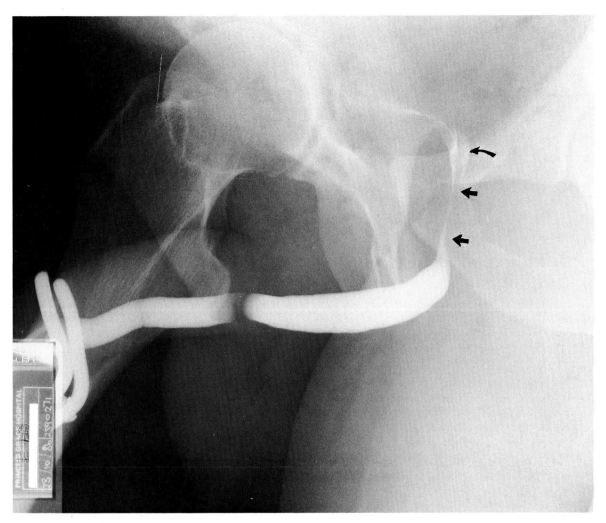

Fig. 1.7 Normal ascending urethrogram.
The distal sphincter mechanism (between arrows) and verumontanum (curved arrow) can be identified. The prostatic urethra is not distended.

4–5 cm long and passes through the tissue of the prostate gland to the apex of the prostate (Fig. 1.7). The urethra is at its widest and most distensible within the prostate gland. The proximal section of the posterior wall is marked with a ridge called the urethral crest which becomes more prominent in the mid portion of the prostate where it is known as the verumontanum. On the summit of the verumontanum is the prostatic utricle, a blind ending sac, flanked by the openings of the ejaculatory ducts on either side. The 'gutters' on either side of the verumontanum receive the openings of the prostatic ducts.

The urethra continues as the subprostatic urethra extending from the apex of the prostate to the bulb of the penis. The urethral sphincter lies just distal to the verumontanum (Fig. 1.8). It is an indistensible region of approximately 1 cm in length and contains the bulbourethral glands. The ducts from these

glands accompany the urethra and open into the lumen within the penile urethra.

The penile urethra is the longest portion extending from the penile bulb to the external urethral meatus. It is initially dilated to form the intrabulbar fossa but soon narrows to form a transverse slit. As it approaches the glans penis it once again dilates to form the navicular fossa, the final few centimetres forming a vertical slit within the glans itself.

The blood supply of the male urethra

The urethra receives its blood supply from branches of the inferior vesical and internal pudendal artery. Venous drainage occurs via the prostatic venous plexus and internal pudendal vein.

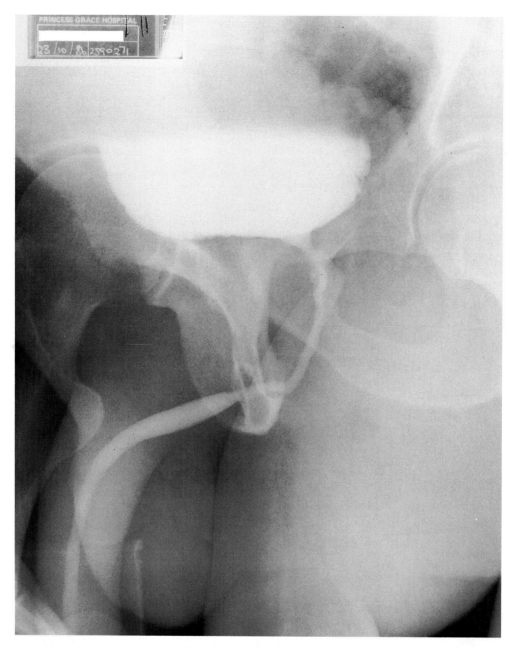

Fig. 1.8 Descending or micturating urethrogram.
The posterior urethra is now distended. The verumontanum can still be identified.

Radiological considerations

The verumontanum provides an invaluable land-mark to both the urologist during endoscopic pro-cedures and to the interventional radiologist when imaging the urethra. It can clearly be seen as a filling defect on the posterior wall of the prostatic urethra on ascending and descending urethrography and marks the proximal position of the urethral sphincter just distal to this. Thus when placing a urethral/ prostatic stent or positioning an intraprostatic bal-loon, the sphincter region can be identified and avoided. Similarly it is important to identify the bladder neck so that long-term prostatic stents do not encroach into the bladder becoming susceptible to encrustation at a later date.

Considerable care is needed when undertaking male catheterization. The prostatic urethra is often much wider than the other parts of the urethra such that catheters may coil up within this section without reaching the bladder via the bladder neck. Force should not be necessary to introduce a catheter and overzealous attempts at catheterization often result in urethral damage, the formation of false passages and risk of later stricture formation. Occasionally the catheter may be held up at the level of the urethral sphincter due to inadequate local anaesthesia and/or muscle spasm. Once again it is safer to abandon the procedure rather than cause long-term urethral damage due to excessive force.

THE FEMALE URETHRA

The female urethra is less complex than its counterpart in the male extending for a distance of 3–4 cm from the bladder neck to the external urethral meatus. As it passes through the deep perineal pouch it is surrounded by the urethral sphincter muscle. The external urethral meatus opens into the vestibule in the form of a vertical slit with prominent surface margins.

PROSTATE ANATOMY

Lowsley's description of the prostate as a gland of five lobes has been superceded by McNeal's concept of zonal anatomy. Three glandular zones (peripheral, central and transitional) and one nonglandular zone (fibromuscular stroma) can be identified on transrectal ultrasound (Fig. 1.9) and magnetic resonance imaging. Normally, the transitional zone accounts for 5% of prostate volume, is located around the proximal posterior urethra and its ducts run parallel to the urethra to emerge proximal to the distal sphincter mechanism. Calcification within these ducts form the boundary at endoscopic resection, the surgical capsule. It is within this zone that hyperplasia and 10% of cancers develop. The central zone accounts for 25% of normal glandular tissue, is cone-shaped narrowing at its apex near the verumontanum. Where the ducts of the vas deferens and seminal vesicles join to form the ejaculatory ducts which then pass through the central zone, there is an absence of capsule through which tumours can readily extend. Five to 10% of cancers originate in the central zone. The peripheral zone constitutes 70% of normal glandular tissue. It envelopes the other zones to form the posterolateral and apical parts of the prostate and is the site of origin of 70% of cancers. At

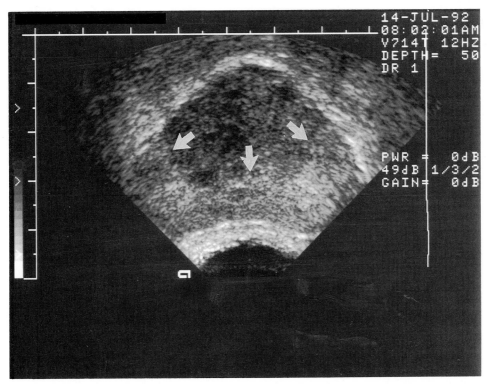

Fig. 1.9 Transverse axial transrectal ultrasound of the prostate showing that the peripheral zone of the gland (arrows) has distinct echo patterns when compared to the rest of the gland.

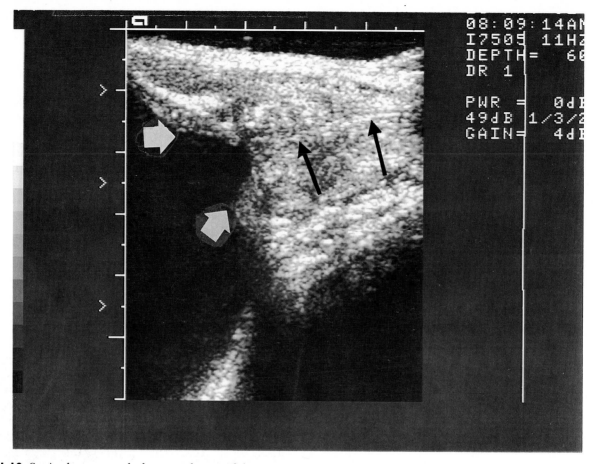

Fig. 1.10 Sagittal transrectal ultrasound scan of the prostate.
The patient has had a transurethral resection of the prostate for outflow obstruction leaving a cavity involving the bladder neck (white arrows). The rest of the prostatic urethra can be identified as an echogenic line (black arrows).

its apex, the prostate capsule is thin or absent and the obliteration of a trapezoid area formed by the peripheral zone proximally, rectourethralis muscle distally and membranous urethra anteriorly indicates extension of tumour beyond the peripheral zone. The anterior portion of the prostate is the nonglandular fibromuscular stroma.

The transitional and central zones are both hypoechoic, heterogeneous and cannot be separated by their tissue characteristics alone, a knowledge of their respective anatomical locations being more important. The peripheral zone is homogeneous and echogenic. In addition, the vas deferens, seminal vesicles, distal ureters and bladder base are well seen. Like transrectal ultrasound, magnetic resonance imaging can delineate zonal anatomy using T2 predominant images using the urethra as a key landmark.

For ultrasound interventional procedures in the prostate gland, the transrectal or intraurethral route is needed. Suprapubic scanning through a full bladder is not able to define the inferior aspect of the gland and does not have the resolution essential for accurate placement of stent, laser probes or thermotherapy fibres. The urethra can be resolved using 7 MHz transducers (Fig. 1.10).

CHAPTER 2

Antegrade pyelography and renal cyst puncture

David Rickards and Simon Jones

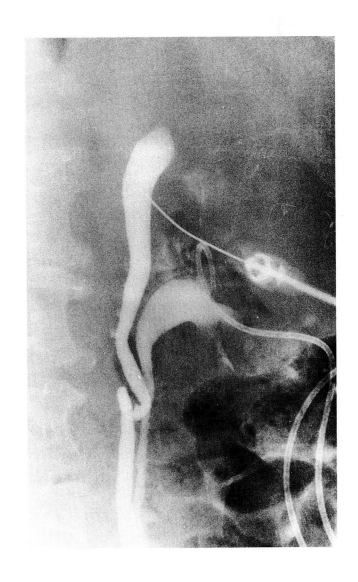

ANTEGRADE PYELOGRAPHY

Antegrade pyelography is the direct percutaneous puncture of the pelvicalyceal system and the subsequent injection of contrast medium. It was first described by Wickbom (1954). Traditionally, retrograde pyelography was the favoured method of directly imaging the pelvicalyceal system and the ureter. Refinements in instrumentation and techniques to localise the collecting system prior to puncture are responsible for antegrade pyelography now being a routine procedure. Indications for antegrade pyelography are shown in Table 2.1.

To identify
1 Level and cause of obstruction to the upper urinary tract*
2 Level and severity of fistulas and leaks in the upper urinary tract*
3 The anatomy of ureteric diversion*

To aspirate
1 Urine for cytology
2 Urine for bacteriology
3 Urine for biochemistry

To measure
1 Resting pelvicalyceal pressure
2 Upper tract urodynamics

To opacify prior to
1 Percutaneous nephrostomy
2 Percutaneous nephrolithotomy
3 Percutaneous tumour ablation
4 Percutaneous pyelolysis
5 Stent insertion
6 Balloon dilation

---

*Where other less invasive techniques have failed.

Table 2.1 *Indications for antegrade pyelography*

The steps involved in antegrade pyelography are:

1 Patient preparation
2 Positioning the patient on a fluoroscopy table with spot film facilities
3 Localization of the collecting system
4 Puncture of the collecting system
5 Measurement of resting pelvic pressure
6 Collection of urine for analysis
7 Injection of contrast medium and documentation of upper tract anatomy

Patient Preparation

Antegrade pyelography is invasive and requires consent. A bleeding diathesis is the only relative contraindication and should be corrected prior to the procedure. Drugs which affect haemostasis are withdrawn. Antibiotics should be given if there is the slightest suspicion that the upper tract is an infected field and continued for 5 days. Premedication is not usually needed in the cooperative patient. The presence of an anaesthetist is essential in the acutely ill patient. General anaesthesia is required in children and the occasional apprehensive adult.

Patient Positioning

For normally sited kidneys, the prone oblique position with the side under question uppermost maintained by wedges beneath the patient's abdomen is ideal. This is a comfortable position. The ipsilateral arm is flexed with the hand by the patient's face. The contralateral arm is by the patient's side. Drips and cannulae are sited in the ipsilateral forearm or wrist. If both upper tracts are to be studied, to avoid moving the patient between doing one side and the other, the prone position can be used with both arms extended. It is not comfortable and not recommended.

Localization of the collecting system

Localization can be done under:

1 Fluoroscopy with reference to a previous excretory urogram
2 Fluoroscopy following injection of intravenous contrast medium to opacify the collecting system
3 Ultrasound guidance
4 Computer tomographic guidance

Blind puncture of the retroperitoneum should not be performed.

The choice depends upon renal function, equipment availability and operator skills. Precise localization is needed in minimally or undilated pelvicalyceal (PC) systems if a first time puncture is to be successful thereby decreasing the complication rate. Puncture after injection of intravenous contrast medium is an attractive method, but if renal function is poor (likely in an obstructed system), it is of no use. Ultrasound (US) is the guidance modality of choice. It provides information on the depth of the kidney, the degree of pelvicalyceal dilation and the position

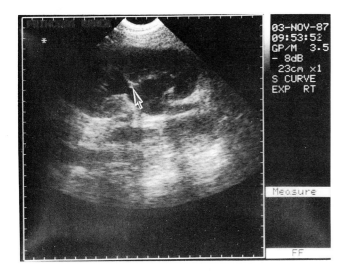

Fig. 2.1 Ultrasound of a moderately dilated pelvicalyceal system.
Under ultrasound control, the needle tip (arrow) can be seen just entering the posterior aspect of the renal pelvis.

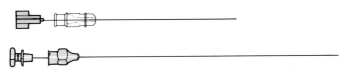

Fig. 2.2 Needles used for antegrade pyelography.
The 22 gauge spinal needle (top) is less flexible than the 22 gauge Chiba needle (bottom).

of vessels in and around the kidney that need to be avoided. Puncture can be done under continuous US guidance to monitor the approach of the needle to the PC system (Fig. 2.1), but asepsis is difficult to maintain. To guarantee an aseptic puncture, US is used to locate the collecting system and the skin marked at a point where a needle can pass clear of the ribs into the PC system in suspended respiration (usually inspiration). The patient's skin is then prepared and the site draped. It is easiest to aim for the most dilated part of the collecting system which is usually the renal pelvis.

In obese patients, or in those whose kidneys cannot be seen with US, computed tomographic (CT) guidance is an option, but it is time consuming and the patient has to moved from CT to a fluoroscopy table if the anatomy needs detailing. The needle is frequently displaced during this manoeuvre and is not recommended.

In those patients who have opaque renal stones and require antegrade pyelography, use the stone as your localization under fluoroscopy. Put the needle tip onto the stone or pass it along the side of the stone. Aspiration of urine may be difficult if the stone is wedged within the PC system.

Puncture of the collecting system

The patient's skin is cleansed and local anaesthesia to the skin and subcutaneous tissues down to the renal capsule is given. No more than 15 ml 1% lignocaine

should be used and if both sides are to be done at the same sitting, 10 ml 1% lignocaine per side is the maximum to avoid the risk of lignocaine intoxication.

Various needles can be used depending on the kidney's depth (Fig 2.2). The 22 gauge, 15 cm flexible needle represents a major advance in interventional techniques (Chiba needle, Cook; DCHN–22–15.0). Because of its flexibility, the shearing forces on the renal parenchyma during respiration are minimized, but such flexibility means that the needle tip is easily deflected from the desired path towards the PC system. Although many passes through the kidney can be made with these needles, each failed access makes further attempts more difficult because of likely bleeding into the collecting system and loss of cooperation and patience by the patient. To this end, the 22 gauge 10 cm spinal needle (Cook; DSN–22–10.0) may be more appropriate as it does not bend as much.

Once the anaesthesia has had time to take effect, the needle is advanced towards the kidney and in suspended respiration, the needle is pushed into the kidney and collecting system. Many operators claim to feel a slight 'give' as the needle enters the collecting system. In practice, with moderately or very dilated systems, there is sufficient latitude that a swift plunge of the needle is less painful than a cautious and slow advance. To see with US the needle tip within the echofree PC system confirms placement, but confirmation by aspiration of urine or pus is easier and definitive. Contrast medium must not be injected to confirm entry. If the needle tip is in renal parenchyma, such a manoeuvre will be painful and may obscure subsequent anatomical detail.

If no urine can be aspirated, it is because:

1 You are not in the PC system. The needle needs to be withdrawn slowly whilst continuously aspirat-

ing with a 5 ml syringe. If that is still unsuccessful, another puncture must be done.

2 You are in the PC system, but the urine is infected and too thick to come up such a small calibre needle. It is likely that either US or the patient's clinical situation will have alerted you to the fact that a pyonephrosis is a possibility. Using an 18 gauge spinal needle for initial puncture is advisable.

Measurement of pelvicalcyeal pressure

A water manometer or pressure transducer records the resting pelvic pressure. Under normal circumstances this should not exceed 10 cm H_2O. A raised pressure suggests continued urine production in the presence of obstruction or reflux from a high-pressure bladder. Normal or low pressures suggest no obstruction or no urine production. Although this step is part of formal antegrade pyelography, in practice it is rarely performed as the information gained is rarely of clinical value.

Collection of urine for analysis

Only 2–3 ml urine are needed and bacteriology is essential. If sepsis complicates antegrade pyelography, knowing the likely causative organism is vital. Cytology and biochemistry of the few millimetres aspirated is useless.

Documentation of upper tract anatomy

Once it has been confirmed that the needle tip is in the collecting system, connect a syringe full of contrast medium through an extension lead that incorporates a two-way tap. It is not recommended that the syringe be attached directly onto the needle. The chance of displacing it is high and it is virtually impossible to screen and inject at the same time without irradiating your fingers. Ideally, a volume of urine should be aspirated before an equal volume is injected. In practice, this will result in needle migration out of the PC system. If infected urine is obviously present, the kidney needs to be drained by percutaneous nephrostomy for a few days first. Antegrade studies in an infected system will result in dissemination of infection and possibly septicaemia. Sufficient contrast medium is injected to opacify the upper tract and define the anatomical problem.

Overdistension will cause flank pain which usually means that the PC system pressure is between 25 and 30 cm H_2O. Spot films of the relevant anatomy are then exposed, checked and, if no further procedures are to be performed, the needle is removed.

COMPLICATIONS

Microscopic haematuria is universal. Flank pain will occur with overdistension (Fig. 2.3), inadvertent injection into the renal parenchyma or perinephric space and injection into an infected system. Infecting an uninfected system is rare, occurring in less than 0.3% of patients. Macroscopic haematuria requiring transfusion has been reported, but suggests poor technique.

TROUBLE SHOOTING

A dry tap

If you are certain that the tip of the collecting needle is within the collecting system, but you cannot aspirate urine, then:

1 You are wrong and the needle tip is outside the collecting system.
2 The urine or the pelvicalyceal contents are too thick to pass up a fine bore needle (e.g. pyonephrosis). A larger needle should be used.
3 The needle has become blocked with blood clot. This usually occurs if you have failed to get into the PC system first time. A gentle flush with 2–3 ml saline should be tried and if the blockage cannot be overcome, a fresh needle will have to be used.

You cannot get into the pelvicalyceal system

This is usually the result of attempting antegrade pyelography in an undistended system. You must give yourself the best chance of success by:

1 Physiologically distending the PC system by opacifying it with intravenous contrast medium and using fluoroscopy for localization.

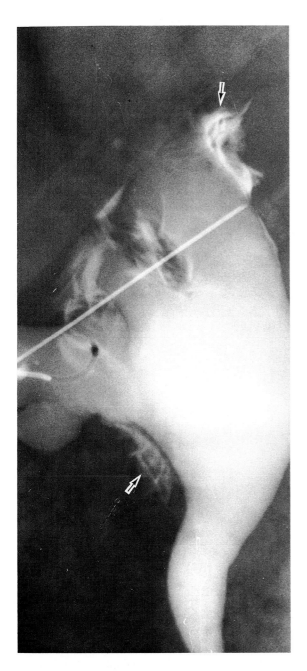

INDICATIONS FOR ANTEGRADE PYELOGRAPHY

If less invasive techniques have failed to document the level and cause of obstruction to the upper tracts, then antegrade or retrograde pyelography is indicated. Retrograde studies require general anaesthesia, but must be considered before antegrade studies if therapeutic retrograde measures, for example, double 'pigtail' stent insertion are planned. The excellent anatomical detail afforded by antegrade studies will usually differentiate luminal (Fig. 2.4) from mural (Fig. 2.5) or extraluminal (Fig. 2.6) causes of obstruction. Leaks and fistulae (Figs 2.7 and 2.8) are usually iatrogenic and well documented by this method. Not all distended systems are obstructed, for example, retroperitoneal fibrosis and vesicoureteric reflux, nor are all undistended systems unobstructed, for example, obstruction in a dehydrated patient. Where doubt of obstruction exists, upper tract urodynamic tests (Whitaker test) need to be done through the antegrade needle.

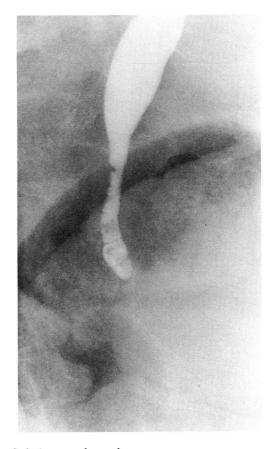

Fig. 2.3 The collecting system has been over-distended at antegrade pyelography and extravasation of contrast medium (arrows) is clearly seen. This will significantly increase the complications of the procedure.

2 Aiming for the most prominent part of the PC system, usually the renal pelvis.

If the above steps still result in failure, it is likely that the PC system will be empty of contrast medium and full of blood due to your attempts. It is wise to stop, send the patient back to the ward and try again the next day.

Fig. 2.4 Antegrade pyelogram.
There are numerous stones in the distal ureter associated with spasm and stricturing of the ureter.

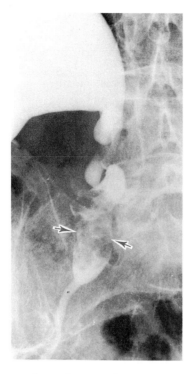

Fig. 2.5 Antegrade pyelogram demonstrating the extent of a large transition cell malignancy in the mid ureter (arrows).

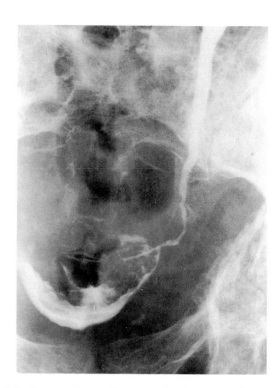

Fig. 2.6 Antegrade pyelogram showing irregularity of the distal ureter due to extrinsic involvement by a rectal tumour.

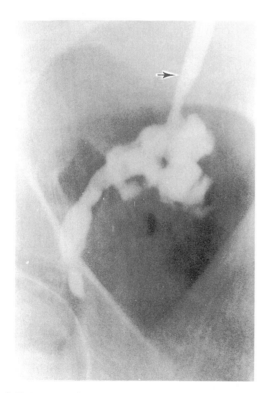

Fig. 2.7 Antegrade pyelogram following rigid ureteroscopy.
There has been complete disruption of the normal ureter (arrow) with extravasation of contrast medium into the periureteric soft tissues.

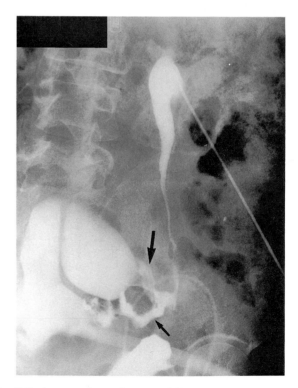

Fig. 2.8 Antegrade pyelogram following abdominal surgery.
There is a fistulous tract between the ureter and colon (arrows).

SPECIAL CASES

Transplant kidneys

Complications of transplant surgery, leaks or obstruction, tend to occur in the early postoperative period and increase morbidity and mortality, so early and accurate diagnosis is important. The approach to the transplant kidney should be a lateral one (Fig. 2.9) as the renal pelvis is usually posteromedial and the kidney is extraperitoneal. This will avoid the vascular pedicle. The superficial position of the transplant allows high-resolution US imaging of the collecting system. Colour Doppler imaging is very useful to ensure that major intrarenal vessels are avoided. Be careful not to overdistend the collecting system as the transplant is denervated and the patient will not report pain.

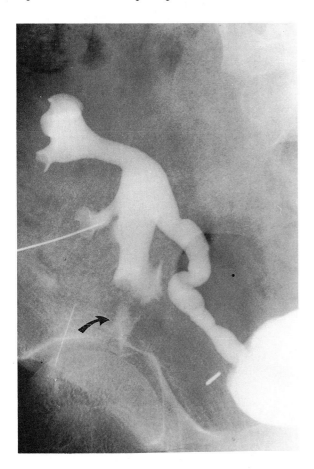

Fig. 2.9 Antegrade pyelogram of a transplant kidney performed because of a persistent leak of urine at the operative sire.
The kidney is not obstructed, but there is extravasation of contrast medium from the lower pole calyx (arrow) due to intraoperative laceration of the kidney.

Postprocedural antegrade studies

Following percutaneous or open procedures to the kidney, drainage tubes are usually left *in situ* to tamponade the percutaneous tract or drain the upper tracts. Before any tubes are removed, antegrade studies should be performed through them to document whether the upper tract is patent with no leaks and whether the primary operative objective has been achieved (Fig. 2.10 a–c).

Antegrade studies in children

These are necessarily more difficult, but the technique is the same. General anaesthesia is essential in all but the most cooperative or listless child.

Ectopic or malrotated kidneys

The upper pole of horseshoe kidneys should be punctured to avoid the medially situated vascular pedicle that occurs in some individuals (Fig. 2.11). Other malrotated kidneys within the normal renal fossa should not present any additional problems. Puncture of the relevant moiety of a duplex collecting system is more difficult as there is less of the PC system to aim for. Pelvic kidneys do present a problem as it is likely that there is overlying bowel which cannot be avoided and a posterior approach is usually not possible because of the bony sacrum. If antegrade pyelography has to be performed in these circumstances, a transenteric approach has to be used with adequate antibiotic cover and by the most experienced operator available.

Duplex kidneys

Both moieties of a duplex or triplex collecting system may have to be punctured to display the anatomy adequately (Fig. 2.12). Should there be a partial duplex with a single vesico-ureteric junction, 'yo-yo reflux' may provide opacification of both moieties by puncture of one of them. Clearly, a knowledge of the renal architecture, if available, before puncture is of great help in planning the procedure.

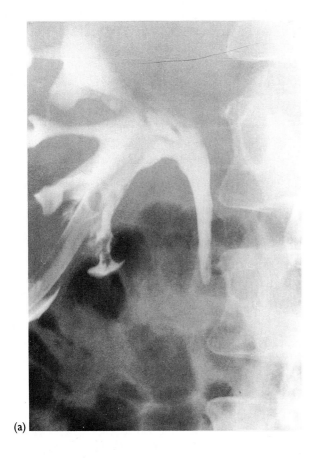

(a)

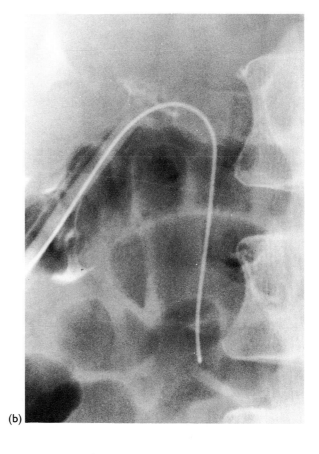

(b)

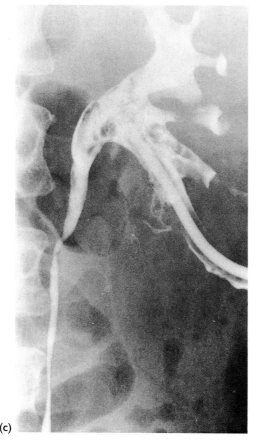

(c)

Fig. 2.10 (a) Antegrade pyelogram (patient prone) following a percutaneous nephrolithotomy. There is a little blood clot seen within the collecting system and an obstruction of the proximal ureter. It was known that the ureter was not obstructed before stone extraction. (b) A guidewire has been inserted through the nephrostomy tube down the ureter past the obstruction. (c) Antegrade (patient supine) following guidewire manipulation shows that the ureter is now patent. It seems likely that the obstruction was due to an organized blood clot or small piece of stone.

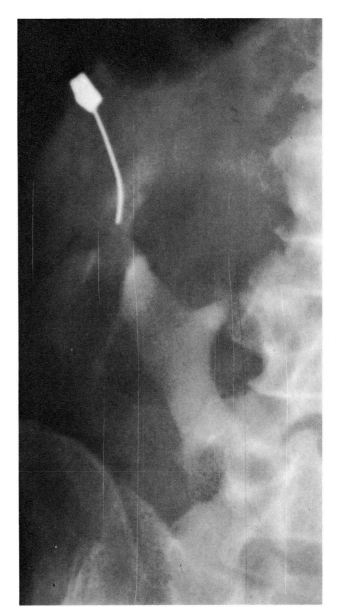

Fig. 2.11 Horseshoe kidney.
The antegrade needle has been directed towards an upper pole calyx which is more laterally situated that the lower pole calyces.

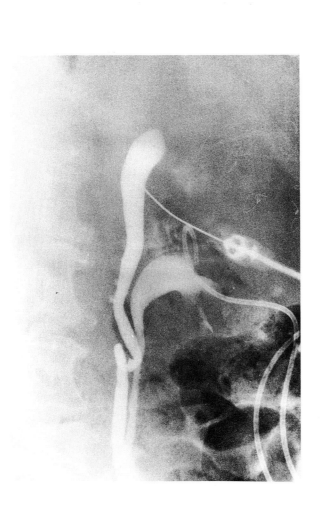

Fig. 2.12 Antegrade pyelogram of the upper moiety of a duplex kidney.
The lower moiety has already been punctured and drained. The obstruction was due to bladder cancer.

RENAL CYST PUNCTURE

Simple renal cysts are very common and rarely require further investigation. Indications for cyst puncture are:

1 Diagnostic
(a) If there is any doubt that it is anything but a simple cyst and that it may harbour malignancy, for example, transitional cell carcinoma. This usually occurs where the cyst is the only possible cause of an otherwise unexplained haematuria.
(b) If there is suspicion that the cyst may be infected. This usually occurs where the cyst is the only possible cause of recurrent urinary tract infections.
2 Therapeutic
(a) If the cyst is so large that it is causing pain or abdominal swelling.
(b) If the cyst is in such a position that it may be partly or wholly responsible for hypertension because it is having a mass effect on the renal artery (the Page kidney). In practice, cysts are rarely responsible for hypertension.
(c) If the patient knows there is a cyst and will not rest easy until it has been aspirated.

TECHNIQUE OF RENAL CYST PUNCTURE

The steps are:

1 Localization of the cyst
2 Puncture and aspiration of the cyst
3 Possible renal cyst ablation

Localization of the cyst

This is best done with US which clearly identifies cysts of all sizes irrespective of their position in the kidney. Fluoroscopy following intravenous contrast medium is an option, but a cumbersome one.

Puncture and aspiration of the cyst

An aseptic technique is crucial and this is best achieved with the benefit of continuous US guidance (Fig. 2.13). The complication of rendering a

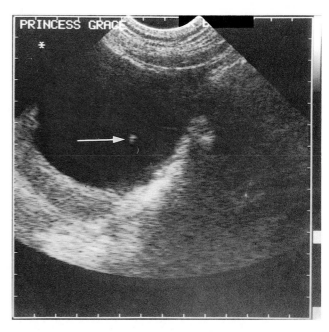

Fig. 2.13 Ultrasound of a large renal cyst showing the needle within the cyst (arrow).

sterile lesion into an infected one must be avoided. Equipment requirements are:

1 10 or 15 cm long 18 or 22 gauge needle (Cook; DCHN–22–15.0, DSN–22–10.0).
2 Connection tubing with an integral two-way or three-way tap.

If the cyst requires puncture for whatever indication, it should be drained to completion. This is easier through a larger bore needle. The length of the needle required can be assessed on US, but it is important to calculate the distance from the skin to the far wall of the cyst, not the near wall. Once the cyst has been entered, connect the needle to a length of tubing with a two-way tap and begin aspirating or, if a diagnostic contrast study is indicated, inject contrast medium and expose relevant views. When aspirating, when the syringe is full, turn the two-way tap off whilst emptying the syringe. This will avoid any air being sucked into the cyst. Aspiration should continue until US has proven that no more fluid is within the cyst (Fig. 2.14 a and b). The needle can then be removed unless a sclerosant is injected.

If malignancy is suspected, all of the renal cyst fluid should be sent to the laboratory with instructions to spin the aspirant down. This will increase the chances of any malignant cells being detected. Sclerosing cysts to achieve permanent obliteration is only a consideration where a symptomatic cyst reforms rapidly and the patient is unwilling to undergo repeated aspirations.

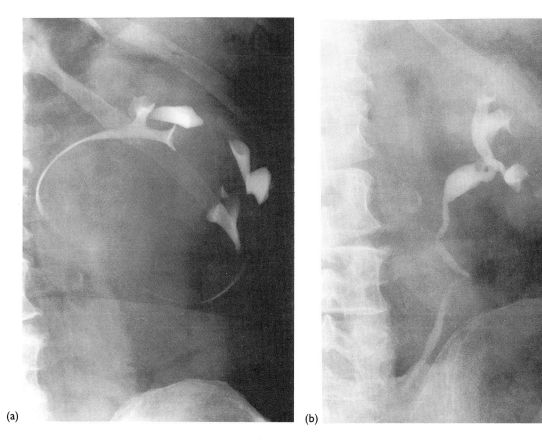

Fig. 2.14 (a) Excretory urogram showing pelvicalyceal displacement due to a large benign renal cyst. This was punctured under ultrasound control and was seen to be fully drained. (b) Excretory urogram, done 1 week after the renal cyst puncture because of suspected renal colic shows a normal collecting system.

COMPLICATIONS OF RENAL CYST PUNCTURE

Haematuria is probable unless the cyst is posterior and the approach to it avoids any renal parenchyma. It is rarely of significance. Infection will occur with poor aseptic technique. With upper pole cysts, a pneumothorax is a possibility.

RENAL CYST ABLATION

For recurrent symptomatic renal cysts, ablation should be considered. This is achieved by aspirating the cyst to completion and then instilling absolute alcohol (95%) into the cyst cavity. The amount varies depending upon the size of the original cyst, but between 10 and 30 ml is usually sufficient. After 20 min, as much of the alcohol that was instilled is removed. The procedure may well have to be repeated more than once. This should not be a routine procedure. It is important to be absolutely confident that there is no communication between the cyst and the collecting system before attempted ablation.

REFERENCES

WICKBOM I (1954) Pyelography after direct puncture of the renal pelvis. *Acta Radiologica* **42**: 505–51.

Suggested further reading

PFISTER RC, YODER IL, NEWHOUSE JH (1981) Percutaneous uroradiological procedures. *Seminars in Roentgenology*, **16**: 135–151.

RICKARDS D (1985) Antegrade pyelography. *In: Obstructive Uropathy*, pp.81–6. Edited by O'Rielly PH. Springer-Verlag, Berlin.

Percutaneous Nephrostomy

David Rickards, Simon Jones and Michael J. Kellett

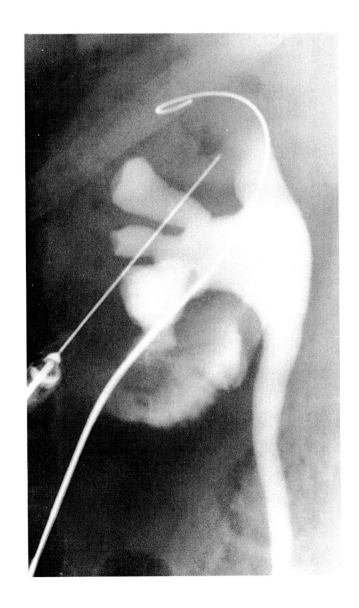

PERCUTANEOUS NEPHROSTOMY

Percutaneous nephrostomy (PCN) has many indications (Table 3.1), but is a predominantly therapeutic procedure to relieve obstruction of the upper urinary tract. The acutely obstructed kidney (Fig. 3.1) will begin to suffer irreversible nephron damage after 6 days. Relief of obstruction will guard against permanent damage and loss of renal function. Percutaneous nephrostomy also provides access for further interventional procedures. These range from percutaneous nephrolithotomy (PCNL) to dilation and stenting of ureteric strictures.

The diagnosis of acute obstruction is not a difficult clinical one, but needs to be confirmed radiologically. Ultrasound including colour Doppler is likely to show a dilated pelvicalyceal system which is adequate enough as a means of localization for PCN. Excretory urography may give more information by detailing the cause, degree and level of obstruction and if delayed films show opacification of a dilated pelvicalcyeal (PC) system, puncture of it under fluoroscopic guidance is performed.

In those with chronic or acute on chronic obstruction, it is likely that the kidney will be smaller than normal and that the PC system may not be very dilated. Puncture is therefore more difficult and localization needs to be accurate.

The majority of acute obstructions are due to ureteric calculi with loin pain and haematuria being the usual presenting symptoms. Most small stones (5 mm or less) will pass spontaneously. Pain is best treated pharmacologically and haematuria can largely be ignored. The decision as to whether an acutely obstructed kidney requires PCN is both clinical and radiological with relative indications differing between centres. If the patient is pyrexial and has loin tenderness, PCN should be performed irrespective of stone size or the degree of proximal dilation as such a symptom complex indicates a pyonephrosis. Conversely, a large ureteric stone with little radiological evidence of obstruction may not require PCN. More definitive therapeutic measures must be performed, for example, extracorporeal short wave lithotripsy, ureteroscopy etc.

Obstruction due to pelvic or retroperitoneal malignancy is a common problem that poses a radiological dilemma. Percutaneous nephrostomy provides a rapid and safe amelioration of impending renal failure that will inevitably accompany such obstruction. It may not be the most appropriate management in patients with disseminated disease.

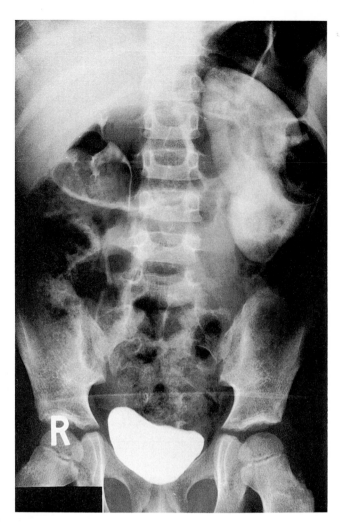

Fig. 3.1 Classic findings of acute obstruction on an excretory urogram.
There is a persistently dense nephrogram in an enlarged kidney and a delayed pyelogram on the left.

Nevertheless, if in the oncologist's opinion the tumour will respond to treatment and it is the patient's desire that PCN should be performed as a palliative procedure, then the radiologist should comply with the request. A unilateral PCN is all that is required in these circumstances. Subsequent double pigtail stenting to achieve internal drainage may be possible.

Leaks and fistulae of the upper tract may well heal with urinary diversion afforded by PCN. Even if healing does not occur, PCN will temporize the situation and permit surgery to be done electively when the patient's condition is considered optimal.

The steps involved are:

1 Patient preparation
2 Patient positioning

3 Localisation of the collecting system
4 Puncture of the collecting system
5 Insertion of a drainage tube within the collecting system

The only relative contraindication to PCN is a bleeding diathesis.

Diagnostic
I To assess individual renal function

Therapeutic
I To relieve obstruction
2 To treat upper urinary tract leaks
3 To treat upper tract urinary fistulas
4 To treat pyonephrosis in the absence of obstruction

Table 3.1 *Indications for percutaneous nephrostomy*

Patient preparation

This is the same as for antegrade pyelography. General anaesthesia should be considered in children and in the potentially complicated case. For the majority of cases, intravenous sedation and analgesia are all that is necessary. This requires patient monitoring. Both pulse oximetry and cardiac monitoring are ideal in this regard. This is an area that has been largely ignored to date, but with the rapid increase in both number and complexity of interventional procedures it is of increasing relevance. Antibiotic cover is essential as infection and obstruction often coexist and infection may be subclinical. Needles that may be pushed through the kidney may enter the colon anteriorly with subsequent contamination of the urinary tract. Assuming the patient has no specific allergies, amoxycillin, 500 mg and gentamicin, 80 mg are given intravenously immediately before the procedure.

Patient positioning

As with antegrade pyelography, for normally sited kidneys the prone–oblique position with the kidney under investigation uppermost is ideal. This allows for manipulation of needles or guidewires under fluoroscopic control without the operators' hands encroaching under the coned beam.

Localization of the collecting system

This can be done using:

1 Antegrade pyelography
2 Retrograde opacification of the collecting system

The technique of localization of the collecting system has been described in Chapter 2. In principle, antegrade pyelography should be performed prior to PCN. The reasons for this are:

1 It permits controlled opacification of the collecting system in an atraumatic manner and this allows for precise puncture of a specific calyx.
2 Diagnostic information regarding the pressure and contents of the collecting system is obtained which may well influence both the approach and technique of subsequent PCN. Antegrade pyelography may not be appropriate in the acutely ill patient who cannot be moved to a fluoroscopic facility.

Because the indications for PCN often involve normally functioning kidneys, the collecting system can be rapidly defined following intravenous injection of contrast medium. This obviates the need for antegrade pyelography even in the acutely obstructed kidney where the delayed pyelogram characteristic of acute obstruction frequently provides sufficient opacification for localization.

Puncture of the collecting system and insertion of nephrostomy tube

Three techniques are available:

1 Modified Seldinger
2 Needle-catheter
3 Trocar-catheter

The antegrade puncture site should be as close as possible to the site where subsequent PCN is likely to be performed. This minimizes the amount of local anaesthesia needed. The site of puncture depends upon the indication for PCN. For simple drainage, the lower pole lateral calyx is preferred. Should PCN precede PCNL or stent insertion, a middle or upper pole calyx is more appropriate. Ideally, puncture should be below the 12th rib to avoid potential damage to the intercostal vessels and nerves and pleural puncture.

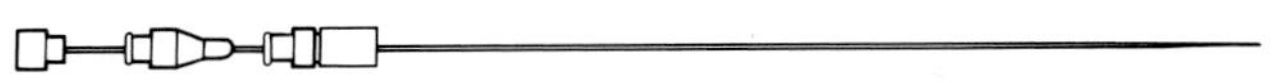

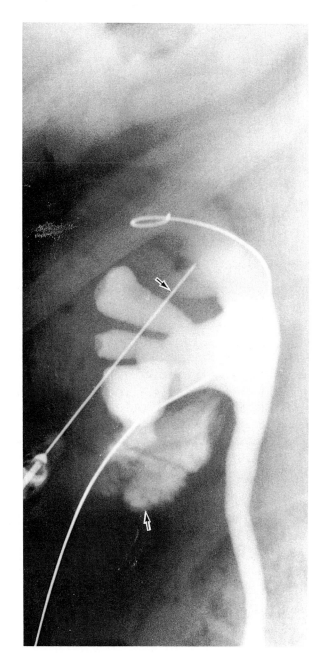

Fig. 3.2a A 19 gauge sheathed needle ideal for percutaneous nephrostomy.
This Kellett needle (Cook) has a diamond shaped tip which is not deflected as it passes through the perinephric tissues in the same way as an oblique-ended needle might.

MODIFIED SELDINGER TECHNIQUE

Once localization has been achieved and the site of puncture identified, a 19 gauge Teflon sheathed needle (Cook; DTVN–5.0–19–15.0–KSR) (Fig. 3.2a) is advanced under intermittent fluoroscopic control towards the appointed calyx. An oblique approach is best to avoid direct irradiation to the operator's hands. The depth of the needle is assessed using parallax by gently rotating the patient a few degrees. Once the needle enters renal substance, its tip will move with the kidney during respiration and the patient should be asked to hold their breath during subsequent manipulation. As the appointed calyx is compressed by the advancing needle, contrast medium within it will be displaced. As the needle tip enters the calyx, characterized by a 'give', contrast medium will re-enter the calyx and surround the needle tip. In all sheathed needle systems, the needle projects slightly further than the sheath itself, so the needle needs to be advanced 3–5 mm more to ensure that the sheath is within the collecting system.

The needle is removed, the sheath left in place and a 0.038 inch 'J' guidewire (Cook; TSCF–38–125–3) inserted until resistance is felt (Fig. 3.2b). Under fluoroscopic control, the guidewire is gently manipulated into the collecting system. Once a few centimetres of wire has been introduced, the sheath is advanced over it to stabilize the sheath within the collecting system. Once this has been done, guidewire exchange is possible if deemed necessary. In many circumstances, the guidewire will pass down the ureter or into the upper pole calyx, should a lower pole calyx have been punctured. In any event, as much guidewire as possible should be advanced into the collecting system. The sheath is then removed and a tract dilated with a fascial dilator (Cook; JCD8.0–38–20) (Fig. 3.3). As a general rule,

Fig. 3.2b Percutaneous nephrostomy.
Following an antegrade puncture of an upper pole calyx under ultrasound control (arrow), the lower pole calyx has preferentially been punctured for nephrostomy and a guidewire inserted into the upper pole calyx. There has been some extravasation around the lower pole (open arrow) which is more likely to occur if the collecting system has been overdistended by antegrade pyelography.

it is important to dilate up to 2 Fr sizes bigger than the drainage catheter because this usually has a self-retaining pigtail configuration which when straightened out increases the diameter of the catheter due to redundancy. There is no point in dilating beyond the site of entry into the collecting system. The choice of

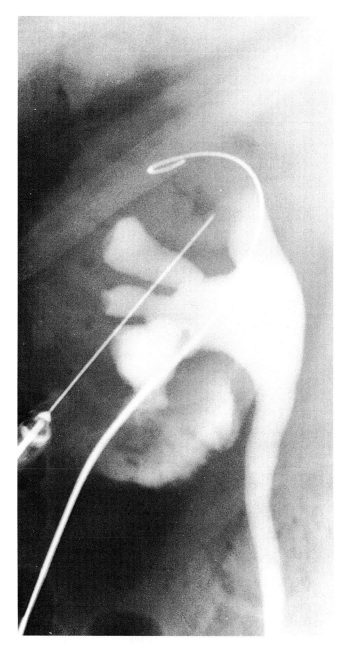

Fig. 3.3 Percutaneous nephrostomy.
An 8 Fr fascial dilator has been passed over the guidewire into the
collecting system. Virtually no resistance should be felt as the dilator
passes through the posterior abdominal wall as the guidewire
assumes a straight line following initial needle puncture, but as the
guidewire enters the lower pole collecting system, it will pass
anteriorly and some resistance to dilation will be felt.

drainage catheters is wide. For draining obstructed,
uninfected upper tracts, a 6.7 Fr pigtail catheter
(Cook; P6.7–38–65–P–12S–PIG) or Cope Loop
(Cook; PU8.5–38–25–P–4S–NCL) will suffice
(Fig. 3.4 a–c). If on puncture, thick pus is found, or if
PCN follows extracorporeal shockwave lithotripsy,

a much larger tube will be needed to drain the system
adequately. Under local anaesthetic, to dilate up to
more than 20 Fr is painful, but can be done. This will
facilitate placing a nephrostomy tube of 18 Fr gauge
(Cook urological; 082918). If only a small catheter is
used, this is passed over the guidewire into the
collecting system whilst holding the guidewire taut.
There should be virtually no resistance to this manoeuvre. If resistence is felt, it may be that the
guidewire is buckling, which is usually at the renal
capsule. If this occurs, the catheter should be removed and the guidewire inspected fluoroscopically
to ensure that it is not kinked. If it is, it will have to be
replaced by passing the initial Teflon sheath back
into the collecting system, removing the kinked
guidewire and substituting it for a new one. If the
catheter ends up in the proximal ureter, it will have
to be withdrawn a little into the renal pelvis. It is not
sensible to leave a pigtail catheter that has not assumed its normal configuration in an undilated ureter. This will cause ureteric damage and subsequent
stricture. Whilst withdrawing the catheter into the
pelvis, rotating the catheter at the same time will
facilitate formation of the catheter's unrestrained
shape. If larger tubes are indicated, an Amplatz
system will have to be used.

NEEDLE-CATHETER TECHNIQUE

This lends itself to acutely ill patients with significantly dilated pelvicalyceal systems. It employs a
catheter over a needle assembly which is advanced
into the collecting system (Cook; HPD–6.0–19.5–
25). The needle is withdrawn and the catheter left *in
situ* (Fig. 3.5). The catheter is preshaped into a pigtail
configuration for stability within the pelvis. The
difficulty with such system is getting all the side
holes of the catheter within the collecting system to
ensure adequate drainage and prevent extravasation.

TROCAR-CATHETER TECHNIQUE

This technique has not gained wide acceptance. In
principle, it involves placing a trocar within the
collecting system and inserting a drainage catheter
through the lumen of the trocar via a cannula.

Irrespective of the technique used, the drainage
catheter needs to be fixed to the skin and attached to a
drainage bag. There are several techniques for this.
We favour a combination of Opsite and Mefix dress-
ings. Silicon discs which encompass the catheter
tightly and are then sutured to the skin are alterna-
tives (Cook; FD–100).

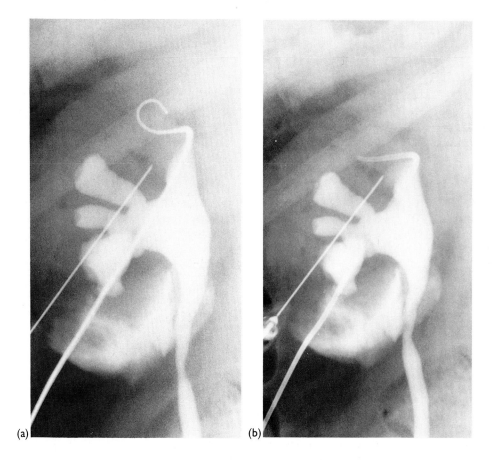

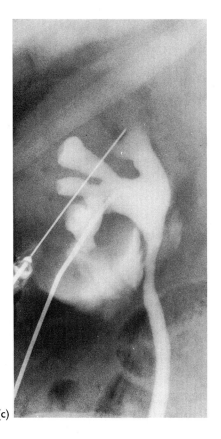

Fig. 3.4 (a) A 6.7 Fr pigtail drainage catheter has been passed over the guidewire into the upper pole calyx. Throughout the procedure, the antegrade needle has been left *in situ* in case any complication in dilation or catheter insertion necessitates reopacification of the collecting system and repuncture. (b) The guidewire has been removed, but the catheter has not assumed it's 'pig tail' configuration because there is insufficient space for it to do so within the upper pole calyx. If left like this and with relief of the obstruction and subsequent collapse of the collecting system, damage to the urothelium of the upper pole calyx may occur with haemorrhage. This may contribute towards poor drainage. (c) To overcome this, the catheter has been slightly withdrawn under fluoroscopic control and rotated at the same time. This has permitted the 'pig tail' to form within the renal pelvis. This is more likely to drain well. In very dilated systems, it is important to leave a lot of catheter within the collecting system so that with subsequent collapse of the collecting system, the catheter does not migrate out of it.

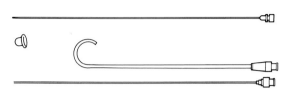

Fig. 3.5 A commercially available needle–catheter kit which includes a needle catheter and stiffening cannula.

COMPLICATIONS

Percutaneous nephrostomy is successful in 98% of patients. Significant complications are unusual and are less than reported following surgical nephrostomy. Complications can be divided into those which are related to the technique itself and those to the catheter.

Haemorrhage, infection and urinomas complicate the technique. Haematuria occurs in all patients, but is usually only transient. The continued drainage of blood-stained urine via the nephrostomy is not of great significance as long as the patient's condition remains stable. If the bleeding is sufficient to block the nephrostomy with clot, it should be irrigated with normal saline or a guidewire passed down the lumen to dislodge the clot. If bleeding is severe and persistent, it suggests that major arterial trauma has occurred and both angiography and embolization may be necessary. Serious vascular trauma occurs in 1–2 % of cases of PCN. Pseudoaneurysmal formation may complicate vascular injury, but can be silent for many years. Surgery is rarely necessary.

Small perinephric haematomas are common and are usually asymptomatic. They tend to be self-limiting and to tamponade themselves. It is advisable to let them resorb without intervention.

In those patients having PCN because of a pyonephrosis, 2% may be complicated by septicaemia. This is more likely to occur if the intra-pelvic pressure is increased by overdistension of the collecting system during opacification and by poor technique. Perinephric abscess may occur requiring

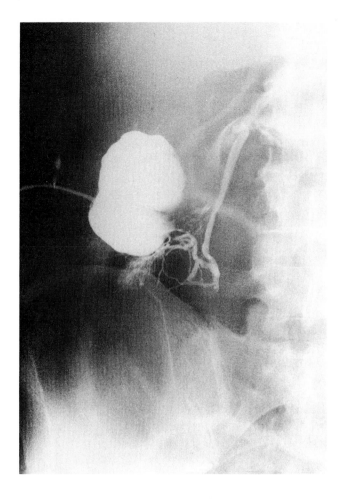

Fig. 3.6 A drainage catheter has migrated out of the collecting system into renal parenchyma and stopped draining urine. An antegrade pyelogram shows contrast medium within renal substance draining into renal veins. This catheter needs to be removed and another inserted.

their own percutaneous drainage. Because the perinephric spaces intercommunicate (see Chapter 1), such infections can involve the whole of the retroperitoneum.

Urinomas are uncommon provided the side holes of the drainage catheter remain within the collecting system. They are reported in up to 2% of patients, but rarely require drainage.

Catheters which stop draining urine are either blocked or have migrated out of the collecting system. If simple flushing does not re-establish free drainage, a nephrostogram needs to be done under fluoroscopic control to identify the problem. Stone or blood clot can obstruct the catheter, especially matrix stone. If a guidewire cannot be passed down the catheter, and should flushing fail, then the whole procedure needs to be done again. Occasionally, catheters may migrate out of the collecting system into the renal parenchyma (Fig. 3.6). Again, the catheter has to be removed and a new one inserted. Catheters can become kinked, especially at the point where they exit from the skin. If simple repositioning fails to resolve the situation, the catheter can be replaced over a guidewire.

Late sequelae of PCN are rare. Cortical scars have been reported, but are not of clinical significance.

SPECIAL CASES

Transplant kidney

The transplant kidney is suited to PCN for the treatment of obstruction or leaks following transplantation. Obstruction to the transplant ureter can be caused by clots or stones, or due to strictures following wound inflammation, rejection or ischaemia. Whatever the cause, if obstruction is thought to play a part in a transplant's decreasing function, it must be relieved as it is an entirely reversible cause of deteriorating renal function. The approach to the kidney must be a lateral one to avoid damage to the transplant vascular pedicle. If leaks occur, PCN is indicated. If possible, the transplant ureter should be catheterized and a draining catheter advanced into the bladder to facilitate both internal and external drainage of urine (Fig. 3.7 a and b). In this circumstance, a single pigtail catheter is used and side holes fashioned along the length of the catheter without allowing its side holes to be extrarenal. Delay in treating such leaks increases the morbidity and mortality of renal transplantation.

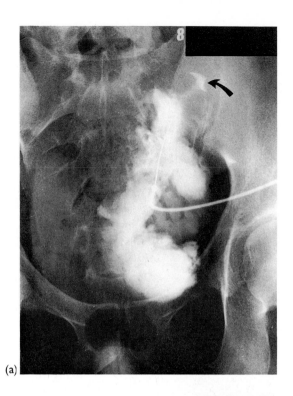

(a)

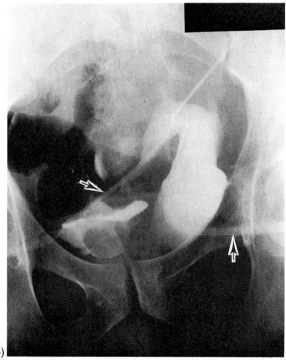

(b)

Fig. 3.7 (a) Transplant percutaneous nephrostomy and stenting. Following transplantation, there was continuous leakage of urine through the wound. Under ultrasound control, the upper pole calyx (arrow) of a decompressed collecting system was punctured and an antegrade pyelogram shows complete dehiscence of the renal pelvis with extravasation. (b) A nephrostomy tube was inserted into the upper pole and down through the transplant ureter into the bladder (arrow). This will provide stabilization of the catheter and so it is less likely to be inadvertently removed. The urinoma was also drained percutaneously (open arrow).

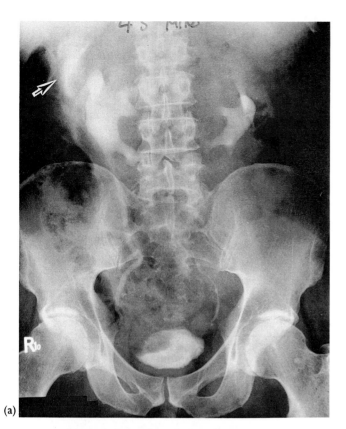

(a)

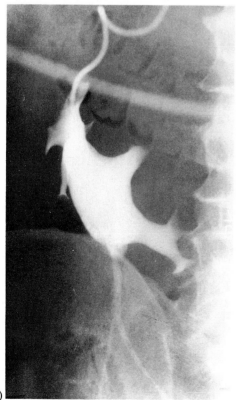

(b)

Fig. 3.8 (a) Acute obstruction of the right moiety of a horsehoe kidney due to a lower uteric calculus has resulted in spontaneous extravasation (arrow). (b) The kidney was drained at percutaneous nephrostomy through an upper pole calyx.

Horseshoe kidney

The upper poles of a horseshoe kidney are more laterally situated than normal and it is advisable to puncture an upper pole calyx directly (Fig. 3.8a and b). This avoids potential damage to the the renal vein and artery which, if laterally situated, would be in the line of a lower or middle caliceal puncture. Clearly, if ultrasound or reference to a previous excretory urogram confirms that the vascular pedicle is medially situated, a lower pole puncture is possible.

Duplex kidneys

The upper moiety of a duplex kidney is preferentially associated with obstruction. Precise knowledge of the anatomy of the kidney is advisable before any interventional procedure. Upper pole punctures in these circumstances run the risk of pleural and adrenal damage and usually necessitate an intercostal approach. When drainage is clinically indicated, the approach to the upper pole must be precisely planned and good localization and technique essential. In practice, a vertical and more medial approach to the upper pole is advisable.

Children

The basic technique remains the same as for adults. General anaesthesia is essential. A prone or prone–oblique approach under ultrasound guidance is the method of choice using a modified Seldinger technique. The French gauge and needle assembly is dependent upon the age of the child.

TROUBLE SHOOTING

Inability to manipulate guidewire down the ureter

The more guidewire that can be introduced into the collecting system, the better. This involves trying to manipulate the guidewire down the ureter, which is not always possible or preferable if there is an obstructing lesion in the proximal ureter. Following a lower pole puncture, the guidewire may preferentially pass into the upper pole calyx. To solve this

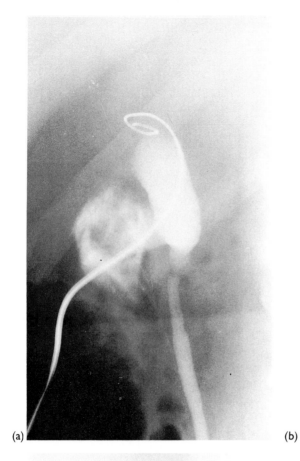

(a)

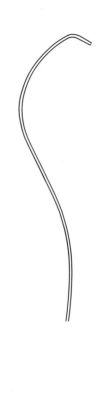

(b)

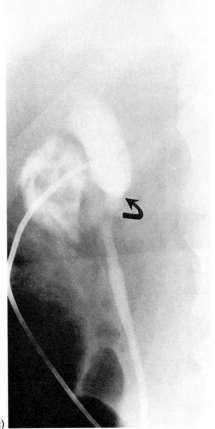

(c)

Fig. 3.9 (a) Following a lower pole puncture, the guidewire has passed preferentially into an upper pole calyx. (b) A cobra catheter which has the ideal configuration if it is considered important to manipulate the guidewire down the ureter. (c) The cobra catheter was inserted over the guidewire into the upper pole calyx, slightly withdrawn with rotation of the catheter until the end of the catheter is directed inferiorly down the ureter (arrow). A straight guidewire can then be passed through the cobra down the ureter.

problem, leave the guidewire in the upper pole calyx and dilate a track to 8 Fr. Then pass a cobra catheter (Cook; HNB–5.0–38–65–P–NS–C2) over the guidewire into the upper pole. Withdraw the guidewire into the catheter and gentle withdraw the catheter under fluoroscopy whilst rotating it. The tip of the cobra catheter will then point down the ureter (Fig. 3.9 a–c). Change the 'J' guidewire for a straight one (Cook; TSF–38–125) and pass that through the cobra catheter down the ureter into the bladder.

Kinked guidewire

It is hopeless to try and dilate up a tract over a kinked guidewire. All that will happen is that the dilator will get snagged at the kink and further advance of the dilator will result in what guidewire is within the collecting system being pulled out. The only catheter pliable enough to pass over a significant kink is the teflon sheath of the original 19 Fr gauge needle used for puncture. Pass that over the guidewire, remove it and replace it with a new one. Should it not be possible to pass a guidewire down the ureter, the use of stiffer, but flexible guidewires into the upper pole should be considered. Very stiff Lunderquist wires should be avoided because of the damage they can create within the kidney should you loose control of them, especially medial rupture of the renal pelvis.

Failure to puncture the collecting system

Assuming localization has been successful, if you fail to puncture the collecting system satisfactorily to allow for guidewire entry, the likelihood is that there will be considerable contrast medium extravasation into the perinephric tissues which obscure the collecting system for further puncture attempts. Such attempts will be further complicated by partial or complete collapse of the collecting system and intrapelvicalyceal bleeding. In these events, abandon the procedure, ensure the patient is adequately hydrated and that antibiotics are administered, and repeat the procedure at least 12 hours later.

SUGGESTED FURTHER READING

PFISTER RC, NEWHOUSE JH (1979) Interventional percutaneous pyeloureteric techniques. *Radiological Clinics of North America* 14: 341–50.

RICKARDS D (1990) Antegrade pyelography and percutaneous nephrostomy. In: *Diagnostic Techniques in Urology*, pp. 119–34. Edited by O'Rielly PH, George NJR, Weiss RM. WB. Saunders, Philadelphia.

SAXTON HM (1981) Percutaneous nephrostomy–technique. *Urological Radiology* 2: 131–9.

CHAPTER 4

Percutaneous Nephrolithotomy

David Rickards and Simon Jones

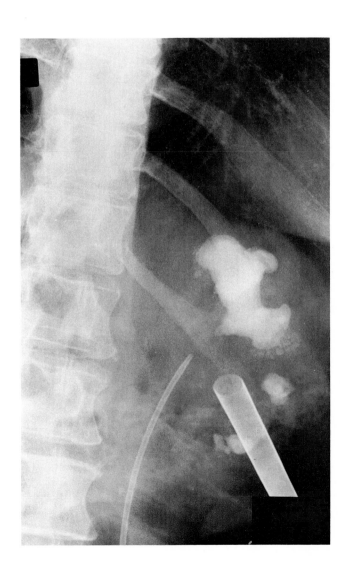

Percutaneous nephrolithotomy (PCNL) was first described by Fernstrom and Johannson (1976) and has since been developed over the last decade by Wickham (1981) and Reddy (1985). Extracorporeal shockwave lithotripsy (ESWL) is now the treatment of choice for the majority of renal and ureteric stones and although it may be the only modality needed, PCNL is still frequently necessary as an adjunct. There are stones that are not amenable to ESWL and are best treated with PCNL.

The major advantage of PCNL over ESWL is that complete stone clearance can be confirmed by direct inspection of the pelvicalyceal system. There is also some recent controversy regarding the efficacy of ESWL.

INDICATIONS

These depend on the availablity of ESWL facilities and inevitably vary upon local practice. Percutaneous nephrolithotomy is favoured over ESWL for:

1 Staghorn calculi
2 Cystine stones and other lucent stones
3 Stones in calyceal diverticula
4 Failed treatment by ESWL, for example, hard stones, inability to focus shockwave due to body habitus, obesity etc
5 Matrix calculi

Localization for ESWL is by biplane fluoroscopy or ultrasound. Machine characteristics will determine which stones are suitable for a particular machine.

TECHNIQUE

The position and size of the stone or stones determines the approach to opacifying the collecting system before puncture and where the puncture is best sited. These decisions are made by the radiologist and urologist together before the procedure is started. Anaesthetic advice must also be sought. The steps involved are:

1 Patient preparation
2 Patient positioning
3 Localization of the collecting system if needed
4 Puncture of the collecting system and guidewire manipulation

5 Serial dilation of a tract
6 Insertion of an Amplatz tube
7 Extraction of the stones
8 Drainage of the collecting system and tamponade of the tract
9 Follow-up nephrostogram and tube removal

Patient preparation

All PCNLs should be done under general anaesthesia. A dedicated interventional suite with piped anaesthetic gases is ideal serviced by a recovery area and a nursing station where sterile trolleys can be prepared. Radiological requirements include a floating and tilting table, an undercouch 'C' arm with a mobile intensifier with spot film facilities. The whole unit must be impervious to irrigation fluids. Ready access to high-quality, real-time ultrasound is useful.

Patient positioning

Initial retrograde catheterization, if appropriate, is performed with the patient supine. For puncture, the prone–oblique position with the kidney under investigation uppermost is standard, as for antegrade pyelography. This allows for easy access along the relatively avascular line (Brodel's line), which lies 1 cm posterior to the lateral aspect of the kidney. Vascular access should be in the ipsilateral arm or wrist. The patient's feet must be protected by soft pads and care must be taken to ensure that any movement of the table top does not impinge on the patient's anatomy. Some anaethetists require that the patient's abdomen be free by bolstering the chest and pelvis. This makes renal access potentially more difficult as the kidney is able to move anteriorly.

Localization of the collecting system

This depends upon the size and position of the stone or stones and the experience of the operator. Various methods should be considered. Some operators prefer puncture under continuous ultrasound guidance onto the stone. This requires experience and if done without the initial passing of a retrograde catheter runs the risk of stone fragments passing down the ureter. Ultrasound guidance has its enthusiasts, but is not recommended.

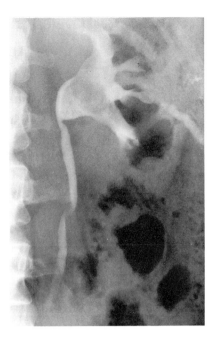

Fig 4.1 Retrograde pyelogram in a patient with a large lucent renal pelvic stone performed immediately prior to percutaneous nephrolithotomy. It was not possible to manipulate the retrograde catheter up the ureter into the renal pelvis in this case.

RENAL PELVIC STONE/PROXIMAL URETERIC STONE

Controlled opacification is achieved by initial retrograde catheterization (Cook; T7.0–35–65–ST–NS–0) at cystoscopy (Fig. 4.1). The tip of the catheter should be positioned in the upper pole calyx, if possible. This is of great benefit to the endoscopist whose orientation within the kidney is facilitated. Contrast medium diluted to 1 in 3 with normal saline and mixed with 2 ml methylene blue to a volume of 20 ml is injected via the retrograde catheter during fluoroscopy. The collecting system must not be over-distended to prevent intravasation. Dilution must be sufficient to allow visualization of the stone.

LOWER POLE STAGHORN CALCULUS

A retrograde catheter is needed to prevent stone fragments passing down the ureter. It is best to puncture directly on to the stone, then to distend the collecting system with saline via the retrograde catheter to create a space between the stone and the urothelial walls. This will permit easier subsequent guidewire manipulation and does not obscure the stone with contrast medium which would make repeated attempts at puncture very difficult (Fig. 4.2).

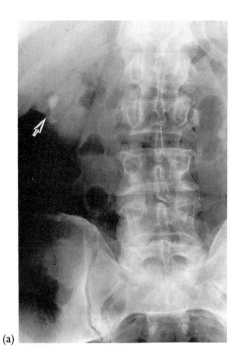

(a)

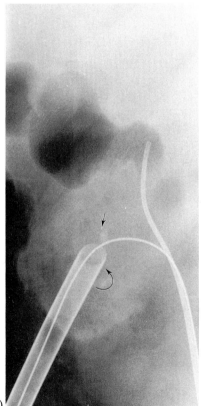

(b)

Fig. 4.2 (a) A plain film showing a lower pole stone that could not be fragmented by extracorporeal shockwave lithotripsy (arrow). (b) At percutaneous nephrolithotomy, the retrograde catheter is positioned in the upper pole calyx which will provide adequate opacification of the collecting system if needed and will prevent small stone fragments passing down the ureter. The guidewire has been left *in situ* during the procedure. A little residual stone still needs to be removed (arrows).

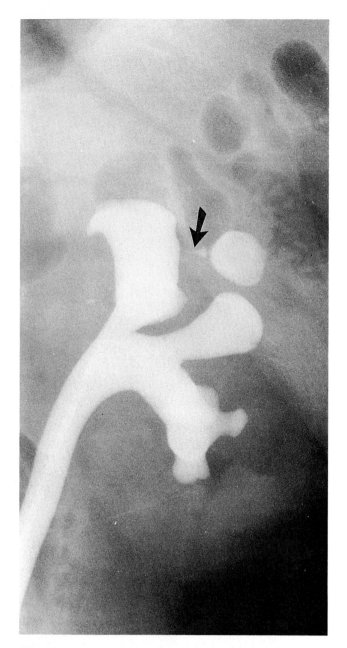

STONES IN CALYCEAL DIVERTICULA

This requires direct puncture onto the stone. It is unlikely that the collecting system medial to the stone will be entered by guidewire manipulation especially with type 1 polar diverticula which classically have a very narrow isthmus with which they communicate with the rest of the collecting system. Type 2 interpolar diverticula tend to be larger and to communicate with the renal pelvis via a broad isthmus through which a guidewire is more likely to pass. A retrograde catheter provides for subsequent visualization of the collecting system should drainage be needed (Fig. 4.3).

UPPER POLE CALCULI

Contrast opacification via a retrograde catheter is advisable. Most upper pole stones can be retrieved through a lower pole puncture.

STAGHORN CALCULI

A retrograde catheter is advisable although the stone itself provides radiological contrast for guidance. The same technique as that used for lower pole staghorn calculi is appropriate. To clear large stones at PCNL may need more than one puncture at more than one sitting (Fig. 4.4 a–d).

Fig. 4.3 Retrograde pyelogram prior to percutaneous nephrolithotomy for this upper pole type 1 calyceal diverticular stone. The diverticulum communicates with the upper pole calyx via a very narrow isthmus (arrow) through which it is very unlikely that a guidewire will pass following direct puncture of the diverticulum. These stones cannot be retrieved via the rest of the collecting system.

Fig. 4.4 (a) To treat this large staghorn calculus, puncture onto the lower pole component of the stone and pass a guidewire down the sheath of the 19 gauge needle. (b) Inject 50 ml saline (which can be mixed with patent blue if required) up the retrograde catheter whilst advancing the guidewire. The distension of the collecting system which this will cause allows for easier manipulation of the guidewire within it. (c) Through the lower pole puncture, most of the renal pelvic and lower pole stone has been removed, but adequate access to the upper pole stone could not be achieved. (d) To clear the upper pole stone, a second puncture directly onto it has been performed in the same way as the lower pole puncture, but the lower pole Amplatz tube was first obstructed by inflating the balloon of a small Foley's catheter within it and then injecting saline either down the Foley's catheter or up the retrograde catheter. The residual calyceal stones were removed percutaneously.

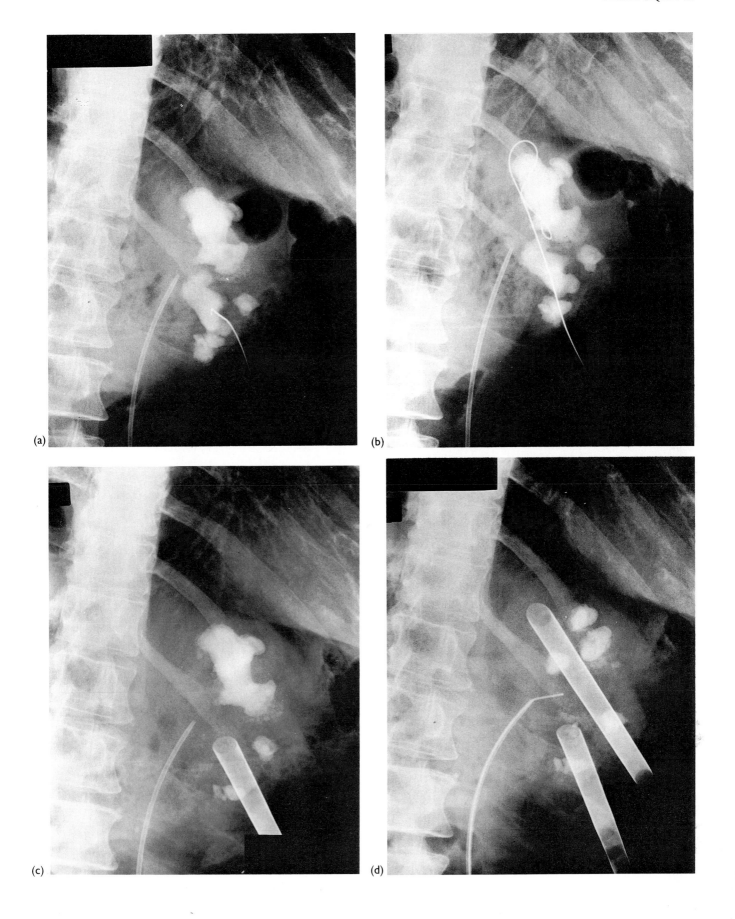

(a)

(b)

(c)

(d)

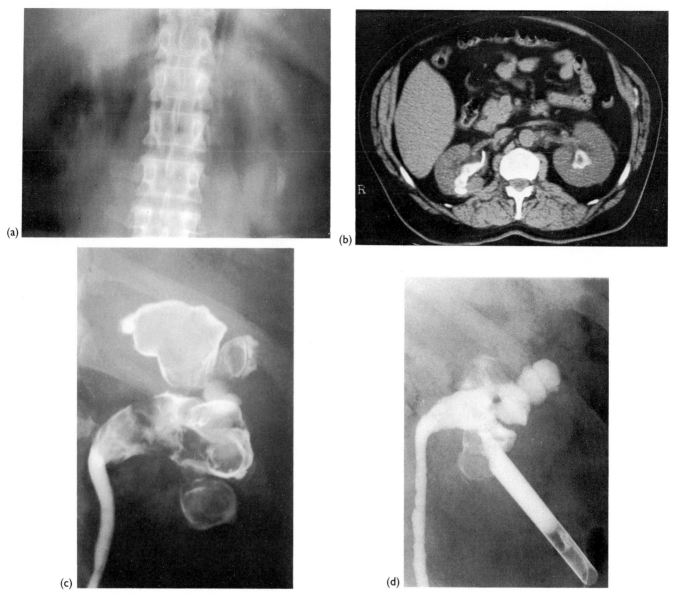

Fig. 4.5 (a) Matrix stone in a diabetic patient in renal failure. No stone mass can be seen on the tomogram. (b) A computed tomographic scan shows the extent of matrix stone within the collecting system. The stone is bilateral. (c) A retrograde study performed before puncture confirms that this matrix stone is filling the entire collecting system. (d) Almost complete clearance has been achieved from a lower pole puncture. Both kidneys were cleared in two separate operations which resulted in considerably improved renal function.

LUCENT STONES AND MATRIX STONES

Irrespective of stone size and location, the collecting system has to be opacified before puncture via a retrograde catheter (Fig. 4.5 a–c).

MIDDLE POLE CALYCEAL STONES

Direct puncture onto the stone without retrograde contrast or puncture just medial to the stone after retrograde opacification of the collecting system are the options. The important point is that any retrograde contrast medium that extravasates either after overdistension or a failed initial puncture will obscure the stone on fluoroscopy making the procedure very difficult, if not impossible.

TRANSPLANT RENAL STONES/STONES IN KIDNEYS AFTER URETERIC REINPLANTATION

Retrograde catheterization is not likely to be possible. In these cases, antegrade pyelography under ultrasound control should be performed which takes the place of controlled opacification via a retrograde catheter. This procedure should also be invoked if the urologist is unable to place a retrograde catheter at cystoscopy.

STONES IN KIDNEYS FOLLOWING URINARY DIVERSION

Stones are more common in patients who have had a urinary diversion, for example, ileal loop, caecocystoplasty etc. Most diversionary procedures are not antireflux. Opacification of the diversionary reservoir results in reflux up the ureters and so controlled opacification is achieved. If this fails, an antegrade pyelogram under ultrasound control will provide the required localization.

Puncture of the collecting system

This is the most important part of the procedure. Subsequent success in removal of stone depends upon it. It cannot be overstressed that puncture needs to be precise and considered. Obviously, the position of the stone within the collecting system dictates the puncture site. In general, the lateral aspect of the collecting system should be punctured using an oblique approach to avoid irradiating the operator's hands. Close control of the sheathed needle (Cook; DTVN–5.0–19–20.0–KSR) immediately adjacent to the skin allows accurate placement. The more lateral approach avoids damage to larger renal vessels.

In a system that's been opacified, as the needle approaches the chosen calyx, it is initially indented displacing contrast medium from it. As soon as it is entered, the calyx refills. The needle needs to be advanced a few millimetres more because the tip of the sheath is not flush with the needle tip. The needle can then be removed and under fluoroscopy, a 0.035 inch 'J' guidewire advanced (Cook; TSCF–35–125–3). Once the guidewire is within the collecting system, the sheath must be advanced over it to allow for guidewire exchange. Ideally, the guidewire should be placed down the ureter alongside the retrograde catheter. With most lower pole punctures, the guidewire will preferentially pass into the upper pole calyx. Although experienced operators can dilate a tract with only a little guidewire within the system, the more in, the better. The tip of the guidewire can be directed down the ureter by passing a shaped catheter, for example, 'cobra' catheter, (Cook; HNB5.0–35–65–P–NS–C2) over the wire (Fig. 4.6), withdrawing the wire into the catheter and rotating the catheter tip into the pelviuretieric junction (PUJ). A straight 0.035 inch wire (Cook; TSF–

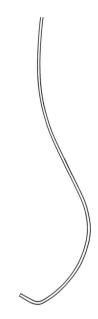

Fig. 4.6 The cobra catheter.
The preformed shape of this catheter is ideal for aiding guidewire manipulation within the kidney.

35–125) is then exchanged and passed down the ureter and the catheter withdrawn.

Direct punctures onto calyceal or staghorn calculi are not always rewarded with guidewire entry into the collecting system. Once the needle tip is on the stone, confirmed by feeling the stone at the end of the needle or with rotation of the patient, a 'J' guide should be passed in the hope that it will go somewhere. If it doesn't, then the needle tip is passed beyond the stone, either superior or inferior to it and a guidewire positioned in the perinephric space.

Serial dilation

This is achieved with serial fascial or telescopic metal dilators (Fig. 4.7). It may be appropriate to use a fascial incisor needle that runs over the guidewire to incise the posterior abdominal wall structures to facilitate further fascial dilation (Cook Urological; 090070). Balloon dilation is an expensive option (Cook Urological; 077030). Fascial dilators carry the disadvantage that the tract is not continuously tamponaded allowing periodic decompression and bleeding into the collecting system. This makes the endoscopist's task more difficult. Fascial dilators are available in kits (Cook Uroligical; 075000), but are also available separately. With experience, dilation can be achieved with 4 Fr steps. Balloon dilation

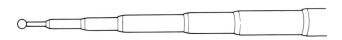

Fig. 4.7 Telescopic metal dilator.
These have the advantage that the tract is constantly tamponaded decreasing the amount of haemorrhage that occurs which would have to be cleared by the endoscopist before stone removal in order that a good view of the collecting system is obtained. This adds time and complications to the procedure.

needs prior fascial dilation to 8 Fr. A maximum of 30 Fr is sufficient. Small stones can be removed through smaller tracts to a minimum of 24 Fr to allow for nephroscopy.

Insertion of Amplatz tube

The Amplatz tube is passed over the last dilator used and its tip position confirmed by fluoroscopy. Once sited, the dilator is removed, but the guidewire is left *in situ* until confirmation of intra-pelvicalyceal position is confirmed at nephroscopy.

Extraction of stone

Whilst the endoscopist is performing removal, it is the radiologist's responsibilty to ensure that the Amplatz tube is not inadvertently withdrawn too far so that access is lost. If the guidewire is left *in situ* during stone extraction, repositioning within the collecting system is facilitated. If the stone cannot be removed piecemeal, fragmentation with ultrasound or electrohydraulic lithotripsy is performed. Stones can also be removed using stone baskets under fluoroscopic control through the Amplatz tube. An angled sheath through which an atraumatic basket can be passed is ideal (Cook; WNSB–12–24).

Drainage of the collecting system and tamponade of the tract

Following stone removal, the tract should be tamponaded with a Porges tube of diameter 2 Fr less than

the Amplatz. The Amplatz can then safely be removed. To stabilize the drainage tube, especially if further interventional procedures down the tract are envisaged, it is advisable to pass coaxially a straight catheter through the lumen of the tube down the ureter. This is easy if the initial guidewire has been left *in situ* down the ureter.

COMPLICATIONS

Percutaneous nephrolithotomy is always complicated by haematuria, but major complications, specifically bleeding requiring transfusion, can be expected in up to 12% of cases. Infection, retained stone fragments (Fig. 4.8) and PUJ stricture are also recognized. With the prevalence of ESWL, percutaneous procedures are more likely in complicated and difficult stones requiring long endoscopy and lithotripsy. Accordingly, complications are likely to be more common.

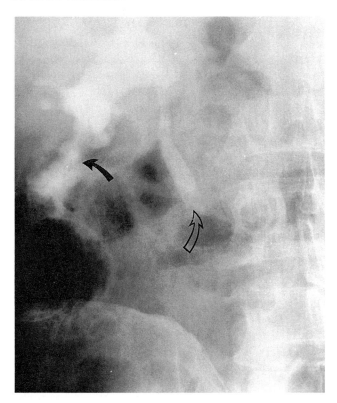

Fig. 4.8 Extravasation following percutaneous nephrolithotomy.
A large renal pelvic stone was removed, the tract was tubed and a check nephrostogram showed an unobstructed ureter. The nephrostomy tube was removed, but 2 days later, the patient leaked urine from his nephrostomy site. An excretory urogram confirms extravasation from the lower pole calyx (the site of puncture) (solid arrow) due to a small piece of stone (open arrow).

TROUBLE SHOOTING

Failure to puncture the collecting system

This is virtually always due to a combination of poor patient positioning and poor technique. The commonest error is to puncture too deep. As a rule of thumb, if the position of the needle tip is in doubt when related to a specific calyx, it has gone beyond it. Withdraw the needle and start again using a shallower approach.

Guidewire problems

It is always tempting to use as a stiff wire as possible over which to dilate a tract. Stiff guidewires have their problems, especially if assured entrance into the collecting system is not possible. Stiff guidewires easily dissect renal parenchyma and when placed down the ureter, can split it. With experience, it is always possible to dilate up a tract over a standard 0.035 inch guidewire. If a wire becomes kinked during dilation, it must be replaced. To achieve this, the initial puncture sheath is reinserted. It is pliable enough to pass around a right angled kink.

Loss of position during endoscopy

If a safety wire is *in situ*, this does not present a problem. Passing a large dilator through the Amplatz over it and reestablishing the tract will resolve the situation. If no safety wire is in place, the procedure may have to be abandoned because any retrograde contrast medium injection will inevitably result in perinephric extravasation. In such circumstances, what is left of the tract should be tamponaded.

Haemorrhage

Haemorrhage is usual when dealing with staghorn calculi because it is not possible to tamponade the transcortical tract with the Amplatz tube. Once some of the staghorn calculi has been removed, the Amplatz can be advanced into the collecting system and haemorrhage will be reduced. If there is too much haemorrhage to allow safe endoscopy, the procedure must be terminated, the tract tubed and the operation repeated down the same tract 2–3 days later. Major haemorrhage that persists may require transfusion and very occasionally angiography and embolization of the bleeding vessel. Haemorrhage is always more likely to be a problem when the procedure is prolonged past the time when the endoscopist can see.

Parallel lie

This refers to calyceal stones. The wrong calyx is punctured and despite good dilation, no stone can be seen at endoscopy. The stone is almost certainly in a parallel calyx separated from the end of the endoscope by an intercalyceal wall. The Amplatz must be slightly withdrawn and redirected. The sheathed needle is inserted through the lumen of the Amplatz and a separate puncture onto the stone performed.

Multiple calyceal stones

It is not always possible to get out all the stones through a single tract. Once a stone has been cleared from one part of the collecting system, another can be punctured through the Amplatz to get at more stone. This 'Y' puncture technique does save on dilating another tract through the subcutaneous and perinephric tissues, but is associated with bleeding from the initial nephrotomy site. It does afford clearance of stone from multiple sites in the kidney. Disparate stone not amenable to 'Y' punctures can be dealt with by two or more separate puncture in the same kidney. The complication rate is likely to be increased, but it is a perfectly acceptable option. It is not appropriate to attempt stone removal from both kidneys at the same sitting.

SPECIAL CASES

Horseshoe and ectopic kidney stones

A clear idea of the exact anatomy of the kidney is needed, especially the position of the major vessels leading to it. Colour Doppler ultrasound is useful in planning access in these cases. Stones in horsehoe kidneys are often more easily approached from an upper pole puncture (Fig. 4.9 a–c).

Transplant kidneys and children

The technique is exactly the same as for that used in normally sited adults kidneys.

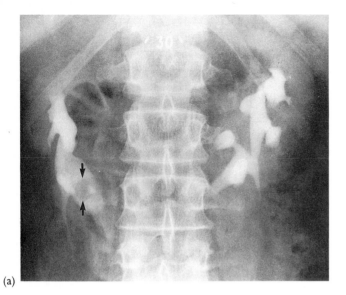

(a)

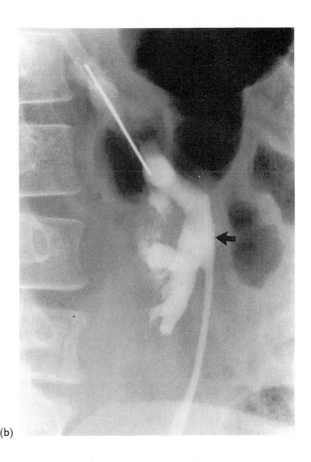

(b)

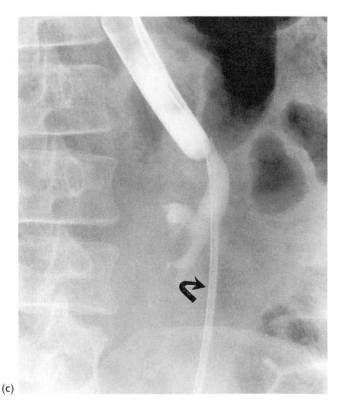

(c)

Fig. 4.9 (a) There is a stone in the renal pelvis of the right moeity of this horseshoe kidney (arrows). The lower poles are medially situated making puncture of them hazardous because of the proximity of major vessels. The ureters are directed laterally and direct puncture of the renal pelvis should not be performed. The upper poles are laterally placed. (b) The upper pole calyx has been punctured after opacification of the collecting system via a retrograde (arrow). An approach beneath the twelfth rib was possible. (c) A guidewire was placed down the ureter alongside the retrograde catheter and the stone removed. Note the free flow of contrast medium within the Amplatz tube.

REFERENCES

FERNSTROM I, JOHANSSON B (1976) Percutaneous pyelolithotomy. A new extraction complete. *Scandanavian Journal of Urology and Nephrology*, **10**: 257–9.

REDDY PK, HULBERT JC, LANG PH et al. (1985) Percutaneous removal of renal and uretic calculi: experience with 400 cases. *Journal of Urology* **134**: 662.

WICKHAM JEA, KELLETT MJ and MULLER RA (1981) Elective percutaneous nephrolithotomy in 50 patients: an analysis of the technique, results and complications. *British Journal of Urology*, **53**: 297–299.

Suggested further reading

LEE WJ, SMITH AD, CUBELLI V, VERNACE FM (1986) Percutaneous nephrolithotomy: analysis of 500 consequetive cases. *Urologic Radiology*, **8**: 61–6.

MAYS NM, CHALLAH S, PATEL S (1988) Clinical comparison of extracorporeal shockwave lithotripsy and percutaneous nephrolithotomy in treating renal calculi. *British Medical Journal*, **297**: 253–261.

CHAPTER 5

Other percutaneous procedures

David Rickards and Simon Jones

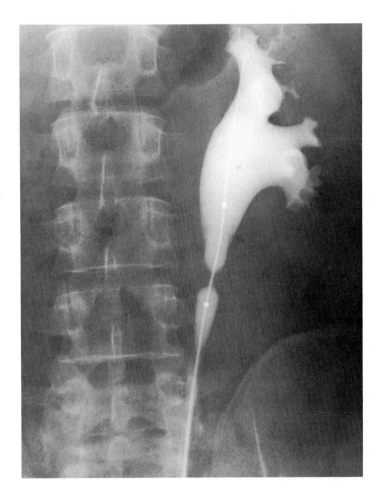

TREATMENT OF PELVIURETERIC JUNCTION OBSTRUCTION

Pelviureteric junction (PUJ) obstruction is usually due to abnormal musculature preventing relaxation. Aberrant vessels as a cause are responsible for 11–18% of cases and they are traditionally treated surgically by Anderson-Hynes dismembered pyeloplasty. Less invasive procedures are gaining ground irrespective of the aetiology. The options are:

1 Percutaneous pyelolysis
2 Percutaneous endopyelotomy
3 Hydrostatic balloon dilation

Percutaneous endopyelotomy

A percutaneous approach to the kidney through a middle or lower pole calyx is established. A tract is dilated to 26 Fr and the PUJ visualized and then incised with a curved cold blade in one place until periureteric fat is visualized. Antegrade balloon dilation using a 4 cm 10 mm balloon (Cook; AXM–6–35–80–10–4.0) is performed to eliminate any residual PUJ narrowing (Fig. 5.1). The PUJ is then stented with a 14–7 Fr catheter for 6–8 weeks (Cook urological; 0077–22).

Hydrostatic balloon dilation

This is performed either through an antegrade or retrograde approach. Antegrade dilatation is performed when combined with other endourological procedures, most commonly nephrolithotomy for stones, or when the ureter cannot be catheterized retrogradely. The steps involved are:

1 Cross the PUJ with a guidewire
2 Place a balloon catheter across the PUJ
3 Dilate the PUJ
4 Stent the PUJ

This procedure must be done under fluoroscopic control under general or spinal anaesthesia and with adequate antibiotic cover.

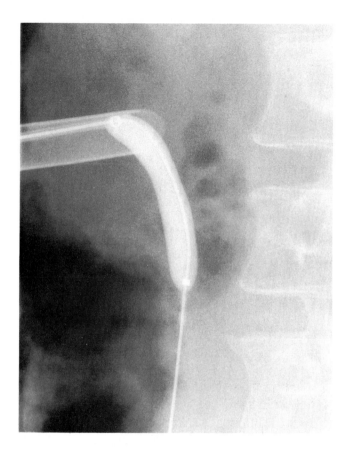

Fig. 5.1 Following a percutaneous nephrolithotomy, an associated pelviureteric junction (PUJ) obstruction was balloon dilated using a 10 mm balloon. It may be difficult to position the balloon across the PUJ such that the obstruction is midway to the balloon and yet the balloon is in a straight line. Overinflation of the balloon will result in it becoming straightened which could damage the ureter.

CROSSING THE PELVIURETERIC JUNCTION WITH A GUIDEWIRE

The PUJ may originate quite high up on the renal pelvis (Fig. 5.2) or the ureter may be redundant, so it is important to determine the exact anatomy by antegrade or retrograde pyeloureterography. With an antegrade approach, the PUJ is located under direct vision and a straight guidewire (Cook; TSF–35–125) is passed through the operating channel of the nephroscope through the PUJ and under fluoroscopic control, down the ureter. When performed retrogradely, the vesicoureteric junction is localized at cystoscopy and a straight 0.035 inch guidewire passed through it and advanced up the ureter across the PUJ into the renal pelvis. In patients with redundant ureters, it may not be possible to pass a straight guidewire. This situation can be solved by:

1 Passing a working catheter over the guidewire into the distal ureter and exchanging the straight

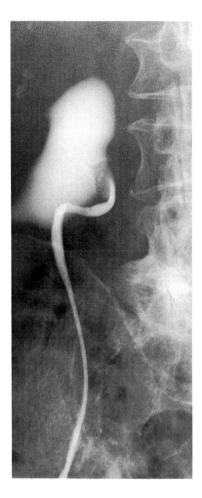

Fig. 5.2 Pelviureteric junction (PUJ) obstruction.
An initial retrograde pyelogram shows that the PUJ is arising from quite high up the medical aspect of the renal pelvis.

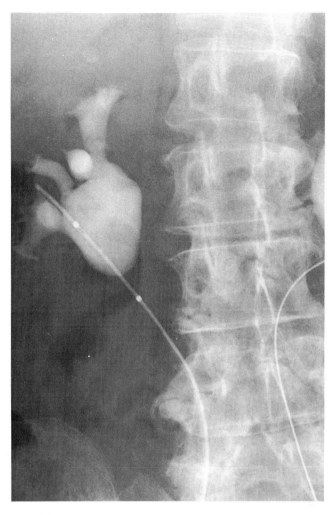

Fig. 5.3 A balloon has been placed across the pelviureteric junction.

guidewire for an 0.035 inch 'J' wire. This may pass preferentially up into the renal pelvis.
2 Passing a cobra 2 catheter (Cook; HNB5.0–35–65–P–NS–C2) over the guidewire and using the inherent shape of it, by rotating it, to negotiate the bends in the ureter.

With these two techniques, there is virtually no ureter which cannot be negotiated.

PLACE A BALLOON CATHETER ACROSS THE PELVIURETERIC JUNCTION

The ideal balloon to use is mounted on a 70 cm catheter and has a balloon 4 cm long which will dilate to 10 mm. Such balloons are available from many manufacturers (Cook; AXM6–35–80–10–4.0). Metallic markers identify the limits of the balloon. This is passed over the guidewire across the PUJ (Fig. 5.3). The balloon is quite stiff and in males, when placed retrogradely, it should be passed through the

obturator of the cystoscope. In females, this is not necessary. With either approach, the renal pelvis should be filled with dilute contrast medium before dilation. When performed retrogradely, this will necessitate removing the guidewire. Once the contrast medium has been instilled, the guidewire must be replaced before dilation.

DILATE THE BALLOON

A 5 ml syringe is filled with a 50:50 mixture of contrast medium and saline. By hand and under fluoroscopic control, the balloon is gently inflated. If the balloon straddles the PUJ, waisting of the expanding balloon will be seen (Fig. 5.4 (a)(b)). If the waisting occurs half way between the metal markers, further dilation can proceed, but if it occurs at the extremities of the balloon, it should be deflated

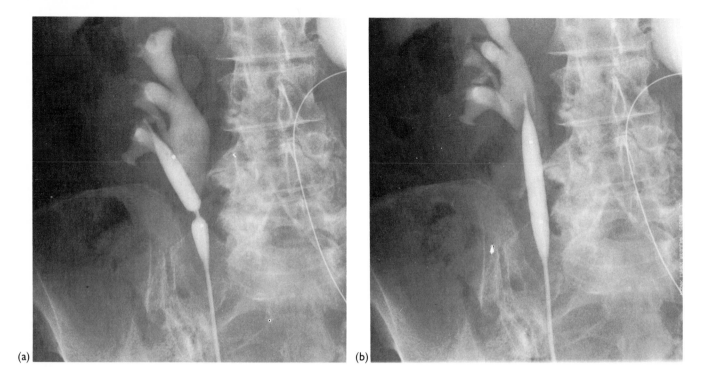

(a)

(b)

Fig. 5.4 (a) The 10 mm balloon has been inflated and the tight pelviureteric junction (PUJ) is well seen. (b) Further inflation of the balloon has resulting in rupture of the tight PUJ.

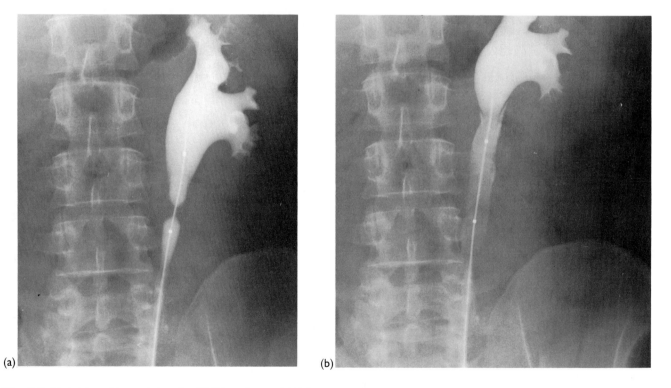

(a)

(b)

Fig. 5.5 (a) A tight pelviureteric junction (PUJ) is well seen. (b) Following dilation, there is extravasation of contrast medium around the proximal ureter. This is to be expected.

RESULTS AND COMPLICATIONS OF HYDROSTATIC PELVIURETERIC JUNCTION OBSTRUCTION

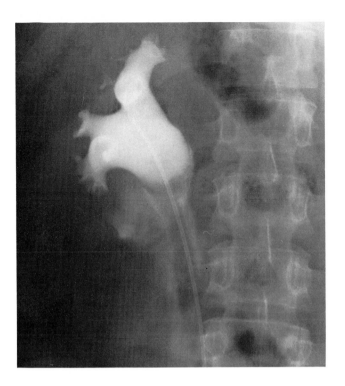

Fig. 5.6 Following dilation and stenting of the pelviureteric junction (PUJ), there is very considerable contrast medium extravasation. This can result in a urinoma which requires percutaneous drainage.

Available series report that this undemanding, cheap and simple procedure is a suitable alternative to open pyeloplasty and percutaneous pyelolysis and is associated with considerably fewer complications. It is indicated in both primary and secondary PUJ obstruction.

Complications are either related to the procedure itself or as a result of the procedure.

1 Patients often complain of loin pain following the operation. This needs to be controlled with adequate analgesia and is due to either rupture of the PUJ and urine leakage into the periureteric tissues or haemorrhage which occurs because vessels around the PUJ have been ruptured as well. This may rarely require embolization.

2 Loss of guidewire position during the procedure. This is potentially serious especially if it occurs after the PUJ has been dilated and ruptures. It may not be possible to manipulate the guidewire either back down or back up the ureter, depending upon the approach used. In either event, the kidney has to be drained by percutaneous nephrostomy which is left in place until nephrostograms show that the PUJ has healed. Without stenting, which is the result if the guidewire position across the PUJ is lost, the PUJ may heal with stricturing. This can be treated with another attempt at dilation.

3 Even with stenting, urinoma formation is possible. It may be painless, but can become infected and be potentially very serious. It is advisable to monitor the extent of the urinoma and only intervene if it is becoming larger, when percutaneous drainage will be required.

4 Pelviureteric junction stricture formation may occur. The PUJ may heal with stricturing which may cause more obstruction that was initially present (Fig. 5.7). Such stricturing may make it difficult to remove the 'double pigtail' stent. In such cases, the options are to try another hydrostatic dilation or proceed to open surgery.

and repositioned. When in the correct position, the shaft of the catheter is stabilized as it may tend to migrate as the balloon is inflated. It does not usually require great pressure within the balloon to rupture the PUJ, but some can be very tight and an inflation device may have to be used. As soon as the PUJ has been dilated, contrast medium extravasation will be seen (Fig. 5.5 (a–b)). The balloon is then fully deflated and removed leaving the guidewire in place across the PUJ.

STENT THE PELVIURETERIC JUNCTION

Because this procedure actually ruptures the PUJ, it has to be stented to avoid urinoma formation. This is done with a standard 6–8 Fr 'double pigtail' stent (Cook urological; Sof-flex 039822) (Fig. 5.6). Large bore stents are not needed and may indeed cause ureteric ischaemia and subsequent stricture formation. The stent is left *in situ* for between 2 and 6 weeks depending upon individual clinical practice.

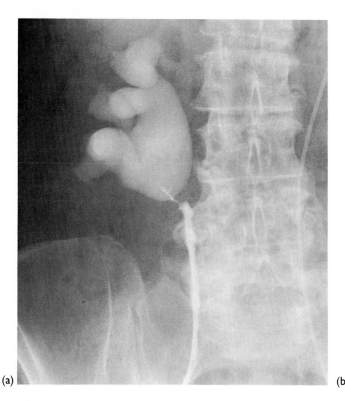

(a)

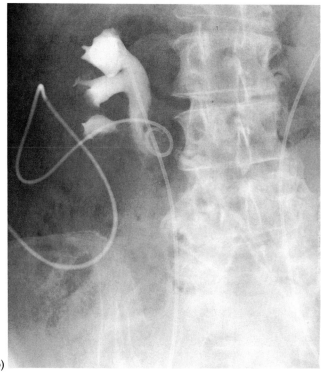

(b)

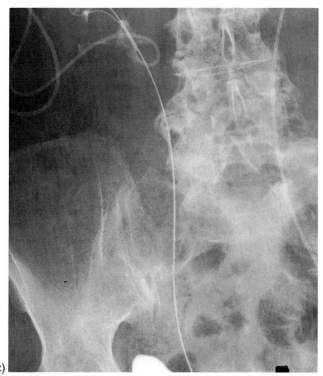

(c)

Fig. 5.7 (a) Pelviureteric junction (PUJ) stricture complicating a PUJ balloon dilation. (b) This complication was initially treated by percutaneous nephrostomy. It was possible 2 weeks later retrogradely to manipulate a guidewire across this stricture. (c) The stricture was stented with a JJ stent. This patient was unhappy to proceed to open pyeloplasty.

PERCUTANEOUS AND URETEROSCOPIC TUMOUR ABLATION

Transitional cell malignancy that involves the upper tracts is traditionally treated by nephroureterectomy. Tumour that involves the bladder is treated by local excision if possible. Local treatment of upper tract malignancy is indicated in:

1 Single kidneys where nephroureterectomy is not an option
2 In patients with poor renal function, where removal of one kidney is likely to lead to renal failure
3 Transplant kidneys where another organ is not available
4 Benign upper tract tumours, for example, fibroepithelial polyp (Fig. 5.8)

Renal pelvic and proximal ureteric tumours can be approached by either an antegrade approach at percutaneous nephroscopy or retrogradely using rigid or flexible ureteroscopes (Fig. 5.9). Distal ureteric tumours require ureteroscopy. Initial preoperative assessment of the upper tracts has to be carefully performed. Focal urothelial malignancy is an expression of field change involving the entire urothelium, so multiple tumours are to be expected. Clearly, minimally invasive tumour ablation is not appropri-

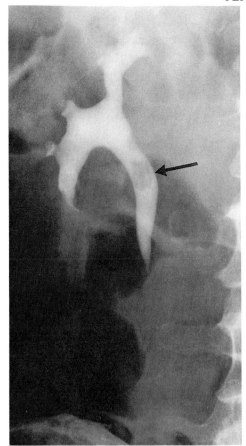

ate where there are multiple tumours in numerous sites, nor is it to be considered where the tumour is evidently advanced and involving either renal parenchyma or peri-ureteric tissue. Once the tumours have been directly visualized, they are ablated with diathermy or coagulated with a neodymium YAG laser. If the tumours are benign, another possibility is to excise them with a cold blade through the operating channel of the nephroscope.

Fig. 5.8 The filling defect in the proximal ureter (arrow) is on a stalk and due to a fibroepithelial polyp. It caused intermittent obstruction and was excised through a percutaneous approach.

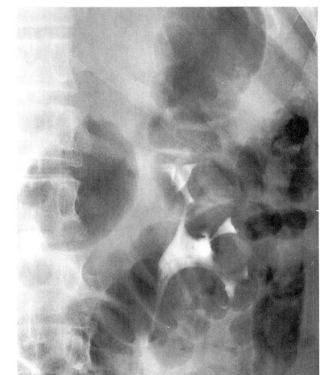

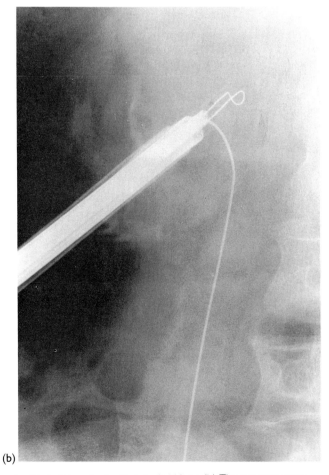

(a)   (b)

Fig. 5.9 (a) There are multiple small transitional cell tumours in the renal pelvis in this patient with a single kidney. (b) The tumours were directly visualized at nephroscopy and ablated with electrocautery.

RESULTS AND COMPLICATIONS OF PERCUTANEOUS OR URETEROSCOPIC TUMOUR ABLATION

In malignant disease, the prognosis for the patient who is considered for this treatment is likely to be poor anyway. However, tumour ablation in the ureter can remove the obstruction in the upper tract and tumour ablation throughout the upper tract can prevent haemorrhage. For these indications, minimally invasive techniques are successful. They are also successful for the treatment of benign upper tract tumours, as long as they are small (the vast majority are) and do not have a broad base with the underlying urothelium (most are pedunculated on a long stalk).

Complications are:

1 Tumour seeding in the percutaneous tract. This is a theoretical complication, but as stated above, the ultimate prognosis in this group of patients is likely to be poor, so the time taken for seeding to be clinically significant is too long. In those patients with a good prognosis, the tract should be irradiated either locally with an yridium wire or with external beam radiotherapy. Consultation with the radiotherapist is mandatory.

2 Rupture of the collecting system or ureter. With any type of upper tract surgery, this is a possibility and is treated by proximal drainage of the upper tract or ureteric stenting.

3 Haemorrhage. This is rarely a problem that requires treatment.

4 Infection. The procedure should be performed under antibiotic cover.

SUGGESTED FURTHER READING

USON AC., COX LAS., LATTIMER JK (1968) Hydronephrosis in infants and children. *Journal of the American Medical Association* **205**: 323–7.

BUSH WH, BRANNEN GE, LEWIS GP (1989) Ureteropelvic junction obstruction: treatment with percutaneous endopyelotomy. *Radiology* **171**: 535–8.

O'FLYNN K, HEHIR M, MCKELVIE G, HUSSEY J, STEYN J (19??) Endoballoon rupture and stenting for pelviureteric junction obstruction: technique and early results. *British Journal of Urology*.

CHAPTER 6

Ureteric Stents

Simon A. V. Holmes, Timothy J. Christmas and David Rickards

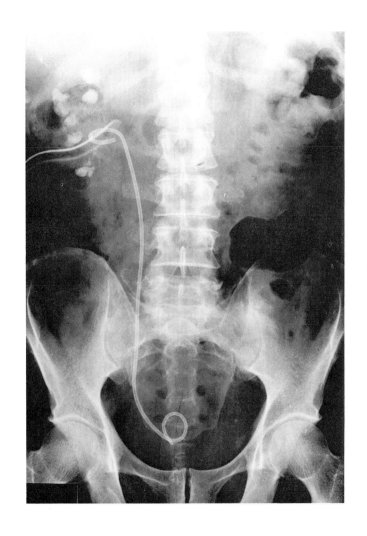

Some innovations in urological practice rapidly gain widespread acceptance through the technical ease with which they can be adopted combined with their demonstrable efficacy and safety. Such an innovation is the use of ureteric stents. The advantages of an internal drainage system over the techniques previously used for upper tract drainage, such as the T-tube or open nephrostomy are appreciated by surgeon and patient alike. The stents can be inserted and removed endoscopically or percutaneously, do not require drainage bags and permit an early hospital discharge. Their introduction has coincided with the revolution in diagnosis and management of urinary tract problems and has helped innovations such as extracorporeal shock wave lithotripsy (ESWL) reach their full potential.

The ureter can also be stented with metallic stents or with catheters that combine internal with external drainage.

INDICATIONS (Table 6.1)

The function of ureteric stents is to facilitate drainage of urine from the renal pelvis into the bladder. They have a therapeutic role as a form of internal urinary diversion, are used as a prophylactic measure to promote healing following a reconstructive operation or can be used as a diagnostic procedure.

The principal use is to provide drainage of the upper tracts across a ureteric or renal pelvic obstruction. Obstruction due to malignant disease which compresses the ureter and causes renal failure can be relieved by stent insertion until tumour shrinkage has been achieved with radiotherapy, chemotherapy or hormonal manipulation. Internal drainage eliminates the need for an external drainage bag and the risk of inadvertent removal and has a lower morbidity than the alternative percutaneous nephrostomy. Such drainage certainly improves the quality of life in patients whose long term prognosis is probably poor. The moral dilemma posed by treating such patients needs full consultation between the oncologist, radiotherapist, radiologist and patient. Whether just one or both kidneys need to be drained depends upon their individual renal function, the clinical status of the patient and the ease with which the stents can be inserted.

In patients with pelviureteric junction obstruction, stent insertion is either a therapeutic manoeuvre by providing upper tract drainage or can be a useful diagnostic tool when cases of marginal

Prophylactic
Lithotripsy of large calculi
Prior to radiotherapy

Therapeutic
1 Malignant obstruction
    Bladder tumours
    Prostate tumours
    Cervical tumours
    Retroperitoneal tumours

2 Benign obstruction
    Tuberculous stricture
    Postradiotherapy
    Retroperitoneal fibrosis
    Stones
    Pelviureteric junction obstruction
    Hydronephrosis of pregnancy

3 Trauma
    Ureteric fistulae
    Postureteric surgery
    Postrenal pelvic surgery

Diagnostic
PUJ obstruction
Loin pain–haematuria syndrome

Table 6.1 *Indications for the use of JJ stents*

obstruction are followed by symptomatic relief after stent insertion. Particular benefits are described in the treatment of retroperitoneal fibrosis in which stents preserve renal function, facilitate ureteric identification during ureterolysis and reduce postoperative complications.

The last decade has seen a revolution in the treatment of urinary tract calculi. Extracorporeal shock-wave lithotripsy, percutaneous nephrolithotomy and ureteroscopy are the principal treatments for renal and ureteric calculi. The safety and efficacy of ESWL has expanded the role of stents as an adjunct to pre- and per-operative treatment. Stone management probably now provides numerically the greatest use of stents with insertion being used to:

1 Relieve acute obstruction from a ureteric or renal pelvic stone
2 Act as an obstructing catheter once a ureteric stone has been pushed back into the collecting system to facilitate ESWL
3 Promote stone fragment passage or relieve ureteric obstruction by fragments

Because ureteric stenting induces dilation of the ureter, stents are used prophylactically in patients with a large renal stone burden (> 25 mm) to encourage antegrade stone passage as the greater the number of fragments generated the greater the incidence of colic and ureteric obstruction. Alternatively, they can be used to treat the complications of stone passage, in particular ureteric obstruction from a steinstrasse. Ureteric stenting is indicated in urolithiasis in pregnancy so that definitive therapy can be deferred until the postpartum period.

The use of stents following surgical procedures, injury or trauma to the ureter has been associated with some controversy, although stents have replaced the T-tube in modern urological surgery. Ureteric stenting causes a loss of normal physiological peristalsis leading to sub-optimal renal drainage. Ureteric healing may thus be facilitated by the addition of upstream drainage with a percutaneous nephrostomy. Percutaneous upper tract drainage can also be achieved with long Porges Bracci tubes, used after lower tract reconstruction or diversion, in which the tubes are passed up the ureters, through the bladder wall and skin to external collection bags.

EQUIPMENT CHOICES

The development of stents in terms of design and material choice has occurred as a gradual progression since the first application of endoscopically placed ureteric stents by Zimskind (1967). The first stents were straight silicon rubber tubes which tended to migrate. Flanges and barbs to promote stabilization were consequently attached, followed by a single and then double pigtail at each end which encouraged stents to remain securely in place. Modern stents are soft with a selfmemory 'J' (or pigtail) at each end which is straightened by insertion of a guidewire through the stent lumen prior to insertion. The stents have multiple side holes, which have been shown to improve urine drainage by up to 40–50%, and markings along their length to aid positioning (Fig. 6.1).

The stents are manufactured by many companies and are produced in a presterilized pack containing the stent, guidewire and a pusher to position the stent in the ureter. The stents are available in a number of sizes (4.5–10 Fr) and lengths (8–30 cm) to accommodate all sizes of ureter in adults and children. They are constructed from various materials including polyethylene, polyurethane, C-flex, sil-

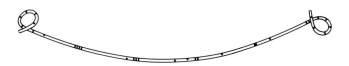

Fig. 6.1 A standard double pigtail stent.
There are multiple side holes at both ends and down the ureteric part of the stent. Markings along the length of the stent assist correct placement.

itek, silicone and more recently hydrogel materials which become slippery on contact with water. This wide range of materials is a reflection of the absence of any single polymer that has the ideal mechanical properties and biocompatibility for prolonged urinary exposure. Silicone is regarded as the most biocompatable, but is soft and more difficult to insert. Polyurethane is stiffer, permitting a tube of thin wall and wide lumen and is thus easier to insert, but is more prone to encrustation and is more likely to cause irritative symptoms. A new percuflex (Meditech 22550) or C-flex (Cook urological; 036622) stent combines the beneficial properties of both (Fig. 6.2).

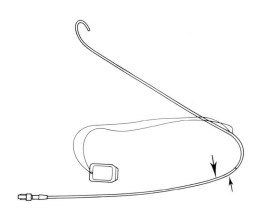

Fig. 6.2 The Meditech stent.
There is a stiffener within the lumen of the stent (small arrow) which can be unlocked from the pusher (large arrow). A suture is threaded through the proximal J of the stent to allow the stent to be pulled back should it be pushed too far into the bladder. Although much easier to insert antegradely because of the internal stiffener, they are a minimum of 8 Fr in size.

STENTS WITH SPECIFIC FUNCTIONS

Lithotripsy stents

Several stents have been produced specifically for use with ESWL.

1 A solid stent with grooved walls that facilitates the passage of the fragments around it, for example, Cook Towers peripheral stent (Cook urological; 037632).
2 A Surgitek Multi–flo silitek stent has large drainage holes, a groove to help stone passage and a monofilament retrieval suture that obviates the need for cystoscopic removal.
3 A large double lumen 10 Fr stent has been produced for stone displacement by Microvasive.

Fistula stent

Manufactured by Cook urological (C-flex 036622–P), the fistula stent has been designed to assist in the management of ureteral fistulae as it has drainage holes only in the pigtails to reduce fluid pressure in the ureter.

Endopyelotomy/pyeloplasty stent

The Cook urological Endopyelotomy Stent (007722) has a widened upper portion of the stent that sits across the pelviureteric junction and holds it open after surgery (Fig. 6.3).

TECHNIQUES OF INSERTION

Irrespective of which technique is used, it is important that the final position of the stent is such that the upper pigtail sits in either the renal pelvis or upper pole calyx and that the lower pigtail just protrudes from the vesicoureteric junction.

Retrograde insertion

If rigid cystoscopy is used, the patient has general anaesthesia, but stent insertion under local anaesthesia is possible with flexible cystoscopes. Fluoroscopy is advisable to ensure correct positioning of both guidewire and stent. Once the ureteric orifice has been identified at cystoscopy, a straight 0.038 inch guidewire (Cook; TSF–38–125) is passed through one of the portals of the cystoscope up the ureter to the renal pelvis. In males, it is easier to insert the stent over the guidewire through the cystoscope under direct vision.

Some stents have a 'closed-end' and need to be mounted onto the end of the guidewire for insertion. The technique is essentially similar using the pusher to advance the stent up the ureter until it is correctly positioned when the guidewire can be removed. Some manufacturers provide stents with a length of silk attached to the distal pigtail which is left passing externally through the urethra (Fig. 6.4) (Cook urological; 036622–T). Such stents can be removed just by pulling on the silk thread which straightens the distal pigtail thus minimizing potential urethral trauma.

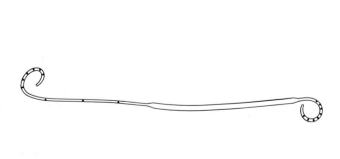

Fig. 6.3 The Cook endopylelotomy stent.
Following endopyelotomy, the wider end of the stent is left across the pelviureteric junction.

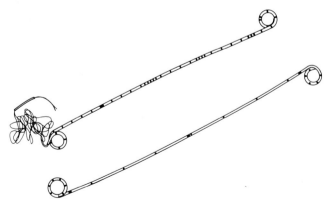

Fig. 6.4 Polyurethane pigtail stents with a suture attached to the distal J to facilitate removal (top).

Antegrade insertion

Antegrade stent insertion is performed:

1 Where retrograde insertion fails
2 Where retrograde insertion is not possible, for example, re-implanted ureter, urinary diversion
3 Following another interventional upper tract procedure, for example, percutaneous nephrolithotomy, percutaneous pyelolysis.

The steps involved are:

1. Percutaneous access to the collecting system, achieved in the standard manner, but a middle or upper pole calyx must be punctured to facilitate stent insertion.
2. A guidewire has to be passed through the pelviureteric junction, down the ureter and into the bladder. The ease with which this can be done depends upon the underlying pathology and the anatomy of the ureter itself. In dilated and tor-

tuous ureters it will not be possible simply to push a guidewire from the pelvicalyceal (PC) system into the bladder and in very distended PC systems, it may be difficult to find the pelviureteric junction. Various techniques are available to get around these problems.

(a) The use of a preshaped catheter. By passing a 'Cobra' catheter (Cook; HNB5.0–35–65–P–NS–C2) into the renal pelvis or proximal ureter, the tip can be deflected by rotation and the guidewire advanced down the ureter (Fig. 6.5a–d). Once the redundancy of the ureter has been negotiated, it usually straightens out.
(b) Negotiating a tight stricture. As a rule of thumb, if contrast medium will pass through a stricture, it is possible to get a guidewire through it. The use of torque-controlled guidewires, low resistance, slippery wires, for example, Terumo wires and small calibre wires (Cook; TSFB–25–145) are all options.

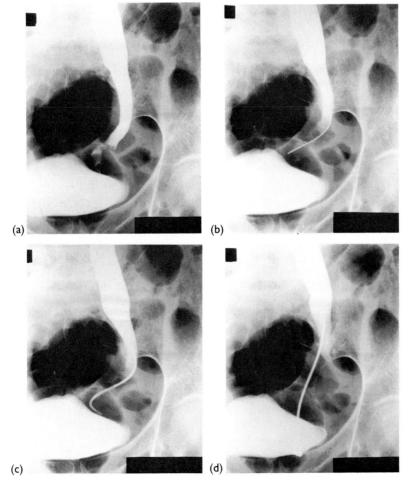

(a)　　(b)
(c)　　(d)

Fig. 6.5 (a) a tight obstructing distal ureteric stricture due to extrinsic involvement of the ureter by pelvic lymphoma. (b) the stricture could not be by-passed with a guidewire because of it's tortuosity. (c) by using a 6 Fr cobra catheter, the tortuosity of the distal ureter could be negotiated. (d) Both guidewire and cobra catheter have been manipulated into the bladder.

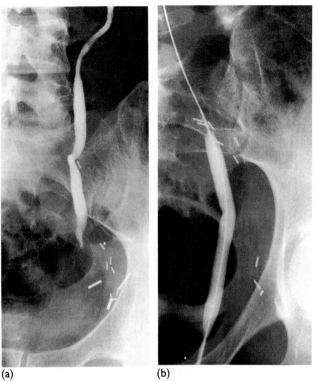

(a)   (b)

Fig. 6.6 (a) A distal ureteric stricture due to irradiation could be bypassed with a guidewire, but not with the stent. (b) A 6 mm balloon catheter could be passed through the stricture because it is a straight catheter and quite stiff, unlike stents. Following balloon dilation, the stricture could be easily bypassed with a JJ stent.

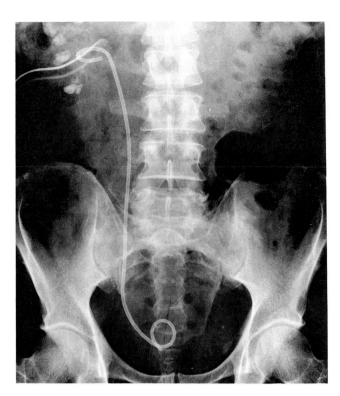

Fig. 6.7 A perfectly positioned JJ stent inserted antegradely following a debulking percutaneous nephrolithotomy for a staghorn calculus.
A Porges tube is left *in situ* tamponading the tract and the stent inserted to facilitate stone passage following extracorporeal shockwave lithotripsy for the residual stone bulk.

(c) Dilating a tight stricture. Once negotiated, it may be essential to dilate up a stricture to allow a stent to pass through it. If the stricture is in the proximal ureter, this can be achieved with fascial dilators. More distal strictures require dilation using ureteric dilators or a 6–8 mm balloon (Cook urological; 010014) (Fig. 6.6a and b).

Once the guidewire position is satisfactory, the working catheter is passed into the bladder and the guidewire used to decide what length stent is needed by withdrawing the guidewire under fluoroscopic control and measuring the length of guidewire between bladder and renal pelvis. To this length must be added a further 5 cm to take account of the pigtails at the stent ends. The guidewire is reinserted, the appropriate stent selected and pushed over the guidewire into the ureter. A pusher is provided in stent packs to push the stent down the ureter into the bladder. The final position of the stent requires that only the 'pigtail' of the distal end of the stent projects from the vesicoureteric junction and that the proximal limb of the stent lies within the renal pelvis or upper pole calyx (Figs. 6.7 and 6.8). The guidewire is then removed whilst the pusher is still in position. The pusher is then removed.

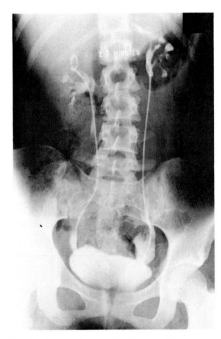

Fig. 6.8 Perfectly positioned bilateral JJ stents.
The right stent is in the upper pole and the left in the renal pelvis. Neither distal end of the stents are in proximity to the trigone of the bladder.

Trouble shooting and complications

FAILURE TO CROSS THE STRICTURE OR FISTULA

In some patients, no amount of manipulation will succeed. Irrespective of the indication for the procedure, the decision to drain the upper tracts having already been made, a nephrostomy will have to be inserted.

FAILURE TO PASS THE STENT DOWN THE URETER INTO THE BLADDER

Although straight working catheters can be passed through the stricture into the bladder, the redundancy afforded by straightening the pigtail of the stent over the guidewire makes this impossible. Options are to dilate the stricture or use special stent kits which allow stents to be deployed through the lumen of large working catheters or stents which have an internal stiffener to them. The latter are large stents, 8 Fr minimum.

PUSHING THE STENT TOO FAR (Fig. 6.9)

If too much of the stent is inserted into the bladder, it will irritate the trigone and produce urinary frequency, potential incontinence and pain. The same situation will prevail if too long a stent is selected. It is not an easy situation to retrieve percutaneously unless snares are used to grab the proximal end of the stent and pull it back. This necessitates another puncture into the collecting system which will significantly increase the complications of the procedure. This problem can be avoided by threading a suture through one of the side holes in the proximal pigtail and in the event that the stent is pushed too far, it can easily be withdrawn. When the stent is in a good position, one limb of the thread is cut, the remaining limb pulled until the thread is totally removed. This carries the attendant danger that a perfectly positioned stent is partially withdrawn out of the collecting system when the suture is removed. This is less likely to happen if the pusher is left in place. The suture cannot be removed whilst the guidewire is still in place.

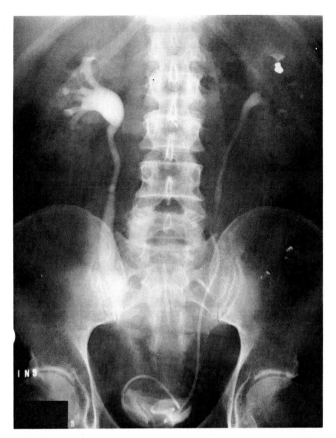

Fig. 6.9 A left JJ stent has been pushed too far and is curled up in the bladder, but is performing it's therapeutic role in unobstructing a distal ureteric stricture. The proximal J has not assumed it's pigtail configuration and if left *in situ* will cause ureteric damage.

NOT PUSHING THE STENT FAR ENOUGH

If percutaneous access has been lost and the distal end of the stent is not in the bladder, it is unlikely that it could be removed cystoscopically as the indication to perform an antegrade procedure was because retrograde insertion was not possible or desirable. The stent may be across the obstructing or other ureteric lesion and could therefore be left *in situ* (Fig. 6.10). Percutaneous removal will then be necessary. If the stent is not fulfilling it's therapeutic role (Fig. 6.11), then a repeat puncture of the collecting system will have to be performed and a tract dilated up to 24 Fr to allow for percutaneous nephroscopic removal of the misplaced stent and insertion of another one.

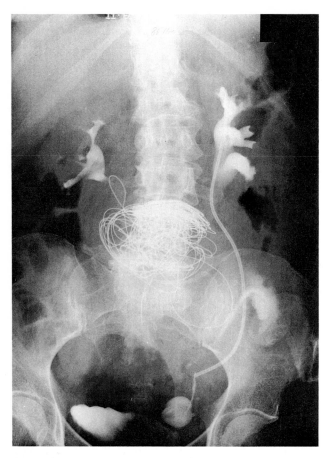

Fig. 6.10 A JJ stent that has not been pushed far enough, but is fulfilling it's therapeutic role. The distal J of the stent has not assumed it's normal configuration. Contrast medium can be seen in the distal ureter on this excretory urogram. The patient had previously undergone surgery for an aortic aneurysm.

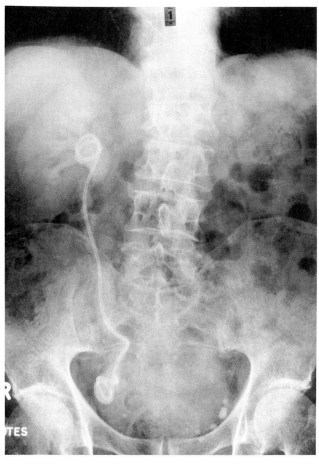

Fig. 6.11 Excretory urogram following antegrade stent insertion for a distal ureteric sticture.
The stent has not been pushed into the bladder, but the stent has assumed it's normal configuration. The stent is not fulfilling it's therapeutic role and had to be removed percutaneously.

PART OF THE PROXIMAL STENT LIES WITHIN THE RENAL PARENCHYMA

This can be complicated by perinephric urinoma formation, but this is rare. It is likely that there will be sufficient side holes lying within the upper tract to ensure adequate drainage. In addition, stents tend to migrate distally on their own.

Combined technique

If retrograde insertion is not possible and an antegrade approach is unfavourable because of poor access to the upper pole calyx (as with a high kidney) or a lower calyx has already been punctured, then a combined antegrade and retrograde technique can be adopted. The guidewire is passed from the site of renal puncture down the ureter until it passes into the

bladder (Fig. 6.12a–d). Here it can be retrieved cystoscopically and delivered through the urethra. The renal end of the guidewire can then be manipulated into the correct position, directed towards an upper pole calyx and the stent can be passed from the lower end into the correct position.

Open insertion

The ureteric stent, by acting as a form of internal drainage, has superseded the T-tube following ureteric surgery. It does not need an external drainage bag and cannot be inadvertently pulled out. Insertion via a ureterotomy is complicated by the fact that a guidewire can not be inserted along the full length of the ureter for the stent to slide over and yet a wire is necessary to prevent the stent uncurling

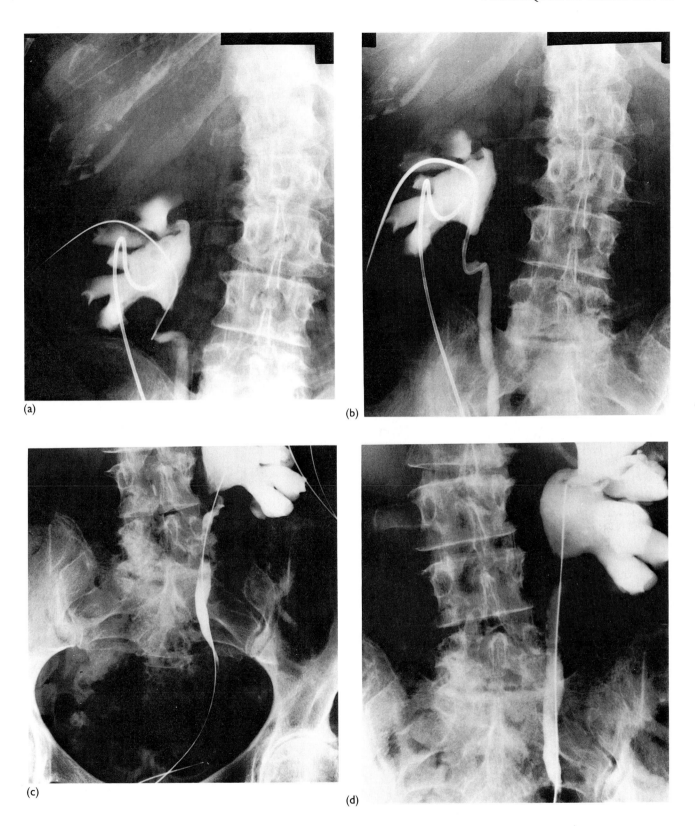

Fig. 6.12 (a) Combined JJ stent insertion in a patient with multiple ureteric strictures. Antegrade stent insertion failed. Through an upper pole antegrade puncture, a guidewire has been inserted into the proximal ureter, but could be passed no further. (b) Using a cobra catheter, the kinks in the proximal ureter were negotiated. (c) The guidewire was passed into the bladder and retrieved cystoscopically. A straight catheter was then passed retrogradely up the ureter over the guidewire, the guidewire withdrawn completely and a new guidewire inserted through the catheter and positioned in a upper pole calyx. (d) A JJ stent was inserted retrogradely and is perfectly positioned in the renal pelvis.

prematurely. The method used is to insert the two ends of the stent separately by passing the guidewire through one of the side drainage holes of the catheter, up the stent and then up the ureter. This is done for each end of the ureters in turn, through the ureterotomy. Percutaneous ureteric drainage is performed after bladder reconstruction with long Bracci tubes passing through the skin, bladder and ureteric orifices.

STENT REMOVAL AND EXCHANGE

This can be achieved by:

1. Retrograde removal with either rigid or flexible cystoscopes. This is the preferred method for stents that are correctly placed. Flexible cystoscopy is performed under local anaesthesia on a day case basis. Stents can either be removed completely having fulfilled their role, or the stent can be partially removed, a guidewire inserted along its lumen into the renal pelvis and a new stent inserted.
2. Retrograde removal with rigid or flexible ureteroscopy. This will be required for misplaced stents where cystoscopic visualization and instrumentation of the vesicoureteric junction is possible.
3. Retrograde removal or exchange with a snare. This technique is for correctly positioned stents and is done under fluoroscopic control under local anaesthesia. The snare, called an 'Angled Wire Loop Retriever' (Cook; AWLR–5.0–50–10) is introduced into the bladder through a working catheter and the stent retrieved. It is an easy technique in females, possible, but more difficult, in the male.
4. Antegrade removal. This will be indicated where misplaced stents cannot be retrieved by the retrograde route and is the last resort, being the most invasive method. If this is to be achieved with a nephroscope, tract dilation to 22 Fr is needed. If snares are to be tried, a working catheter with a lumen of 10 Fr will suffice. The snare can then be passed through the working catheter and the stent retrieved.

SPECIAL CASES

Renal transplants

Renal transplantation will usually involve ureteric implantation of the graft into the host bladder. The majority of transplant units do not routinely use a stent to protect this anastomosis as it is unnecessary and there is evidence that the transplanted ureter fares better without a foreign body inside it. Stents do, however, have an important role in the management of the urological complications of transplant recipients. Obstruction, anastomotic leakage and fistula formation are not uncommon postoperative sequelae which may compromise the graft and the life of the patient in the early postoperative period when high doses of steroids are administered. The stents, which can be inserted in a retrograde or antegrade fashion or at open operation, may obviate the need for any further surgery or may allow postponement of definitive surgical correction until renal function has stabilized and immunosuppression has been reduced.

Urinary diversion

The diversion of urine from the upper renal tracts away from the bladder may be necessary to protect distal suture lines. Long stents are placed in the ureter at open operation and provide external drainage through the skin, the urethra or an ileal or colonic conduit. These stents are sewn in place with an absorbable suture which allows removal after 10 days. An example is the Porges Bracci tube.

COMPLICATIONS

Urinary frequency, dysuria or incontinence

With retrograde insertion, this may be transient and due to cystoscopy. If prolonged or following antegrade insertion it is almost certainly because too long a stent has been used and the distal end of the stent is lying on the patient's trigone and irritating it. Incontinence will further complicate because of urinary infection, secondary detrusor instability or the end of the stent may protrude through the bladder neck. This is a wholly avoidable complication. In practice, 22 or 24 cm stents are sufficient in all but the tallest of patients.

Haematuria

This is usually transient and the result of instrumentation. If prolonged with antegrade insertion, renal vascular damage must be suspected and microscopic haematuria can be expected if infection is present.

Ureteric stricture

This may occur following:

1. Ureteric rupture. Most retrograde stent insertions are performed in theatre without fluoroscopic guidance. In patients with tortuous ureters, obstructing ureteric lesions or pre-existing ureteric stricture, it is inevitable that in some the guidewire will be pushed through the ureter and the stent inserted over it. It is unlikely that a good therapeutic result will occur and the mistake will be quickly diagnosed and rectified. However, the damaged ureter, despite adequate stenting, may heal with fibrosis and subsequent stricture formation (Fig. 6.13).
2. Misplaced stents. If the pigtails of the stent lie within the ureter, it is unlikely that it will assume its preshaped configuration, but it will try to do so and if left *in situ* for too long, ureteric damage resulting in either stricture formation or perforation may occur. Although such misplaced stents may be performing a perfectly adequate therapeutic role and it is tempting to leave them *in situ*, this is bad practice.

Stent migration

Misplaced stents are more likely to migrate than those that are in good a position and are of the correct length. It is more likely that the stent will migrate caudally to lie largely or completely within the bladder. Proximal migration may require nephrostomy for removal.

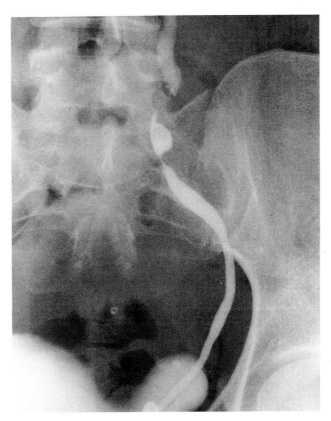

Fig. 6.13 Ureteric stricture complicating JJ stent insertion.

Stent encrustation

Stones can form on the stent or block the lumen of the stent. This is likely to occur in:

1. Stone formers. Pre-existing stones may attach themselves to any part of the stent and stones can form on the stent which acts as a foreign body. Although this is more likely to happen in stents which have been *in situ* for longer than 6 weeks, it can happen within days of the stent being inserted. The patient's previous history and urinary chemistry will alert the clinician to this complication and will advance the time that a stent should be exchanged for a new one (Figs. 6.14 and 6.15).
2. Infected urine. The urease producing organisms such as *Proteus mirabilis* raise the pH of urine so that the solubility product of magnesium ammonium phosphate is exceeded and it precipitates out onto any foreign body in the urinary tract. Large deposits rapidly form which harbour further infecting organisms leading to the development of a vicious cycle (Fig. 6.17).

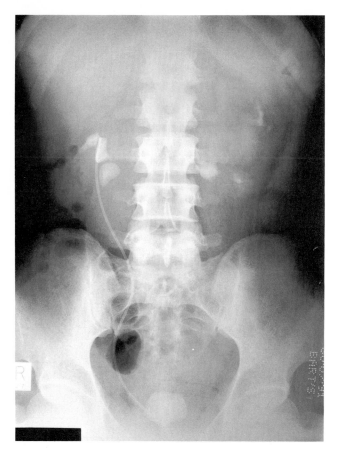

Fig. 6.14 JJ stent inserted prior to extracorporeal shockwave lithotripsy for a small right renal stone in a patient with hyperparathyroidism and bilateral stones. The patient defaulted from treatment and at 5 months there is extensive stone formation around both ends of the stent.

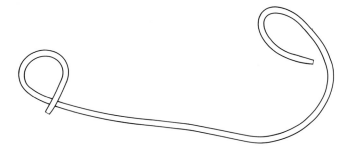

Fig. 6.16 Extensive encrustation along the entire length of a JJ stent which could be removed cystoscopically.

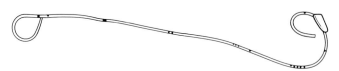

Fig. 6.15 Small stone formed around the lower end of a JJ stent which was removed cystoscopically.

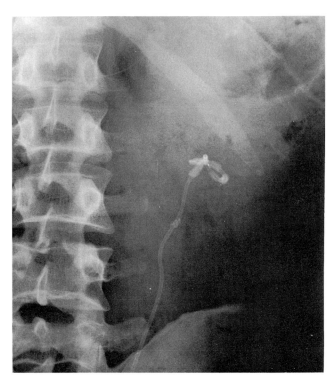

Fig. 6.17 There is stone formation around the upper end of this JJ stent. It could not be removed cystoscopically and had to be retrieved at percutaneous nephroscopy.

Stent fracture

Polyurethane stents, when left *in situ* for long periods of time, become brittle and can fracture spontaneously due to depolymerization by free radical and hydrolytic degradation. The renal fragment will usually require percutaneous retrieval although they have been known to pass spontaneously.

REFERENCES

ZIMSKIND PD, FETTER TR, WILKINSON JL (1967) Clinical use of long-term indwelling silicon rubber ureteral splints inserted endoscopically. *Journal of Urology*, **97**: 840–44.

Suggested Further Reading

PAYNE SR, RAMSAY JWA (1988) The effects of double J stents on renal pelvic dynamics of the pig. *Journal of Urology*. **140**: 637–41.

POCOCK RD, STOWER MJ, FERRO MA, SMITH PJB, GINGELL JC (1986) Double J stents. A review of 100 patients. *British Journal of Urology*. **58**: 629–33.

SALTZMAN B (1988) Ureteral stents. Indications, variations and complications. *Urological Clinics of North America*. **15**: 481–91.

WALMSLEY BH, ABERCROMBIE GF (1987) 'J' stents. *Recent Advances in Urology. IV.* Edited by Hendry WF. Churchill Livingstone, Edinburgh.

CHAPTER 7

Percutaneous Biopsy

Archie Alexander and Matthew D. Rifkin

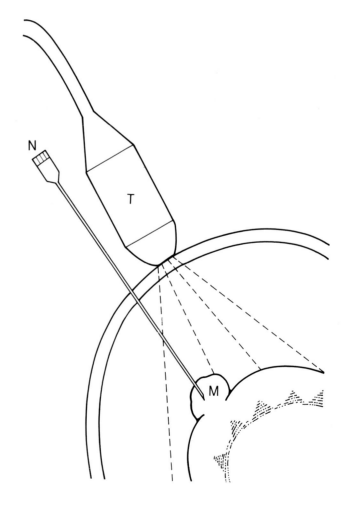

Percutaneous renal biopsy has become instrumental in the early diagnosis of diseases affecting the native kidneys as well as the early assessment of renal allograft dysfunction. In addition, percutaneous sampling of renal masses facilitates differentiation between benign and malignant processes and the diagnosis of infected renal masses such as carbuncles.

EQUIPMENT REQUIREMENTS

The basic equipment needs for renal biopsy are (Fig. 7.1):

1 Several luer lock syringes are needed, volumes ranging from 5 to 10 ml. Much larger syringes (20–60 ml) are reserved for aspirations of thick material
2 A packet of sterile gauze
3 No. 11 scalpel blade
4 Sterile drapes
5 Glass slides
6 Topical sterilizing fluid (alcohol and betadine solution)
7 A vial of local anaesthetic (1% lignocaine)

Selection of the proper needle is critical to the success of percutaneous sampling for renal tissues. Many factors must be considered before the correct gauge, length and type of needle tip are selected. First is the target tissue to be sampled and the type of specimen desired. Specimens are taken for either cytological (cell) or pathological (core specimen) analysis. Next,

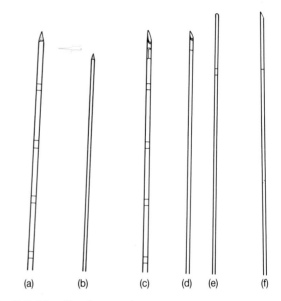

Fig. 7.2 Needles for cytology.
(A) Franseen (18,20 and 22 gauge). (B) Menghini (16,18 and 10 gauge). (C) Westcott (22 and 20 gauge) (D) Spinal needle (20 gauge) (sono-tip). (E) Spinal needle (22 gauge) (sono-tip). (F) Spinal needle (22 gauge) (sono-tip).

some thought should be given to the vascularity of the lesion since a larger gauge needle may increase the risk of significant haemorrhage. Finally, attention is allotted to the imaging device and type of guidance required during the biopsy.

Specimens suitable for a cytological diagnosis are obtained with a fine needle (20–23 gauge), for example, a Chiba or a spinal style needle. If more specimen volume is desired, then a cutting needle is used, for example, a Westcott, Franseen or Menghini needle. Both the Franseen and Westcott needles come in 22 gauge, but the Menghini is a slightly larger 20 gauge. Most of these needles are 15 cm in length which covers the distance from the skin surface to the retroperitoneum and the kidney (Fig. 7.2). To procure a core biopsy specimen, an 18 gauge needle is usually needed. Larger needles should be avoided because of the potential for neoplastic seeding of the tract after biopsy which has been reported with the 14 gauge Vin-Silverman or Franklin-Silverman needle. This risk is much less when aspiration is performed with a fine needle. Experimentally, this difference has been attributed to the reduced number of cells deposited within the tract after the removal of a thin needle. Also, the chance of a significance haemorrhage is increased with large needles. Using 18 gauge needles for core biopsy, the risk is low and has to be considered in the context of a long-term complication in a patient with malignant disease. Currently, many core samples are acquired with an automated, hand-held trigger device con-

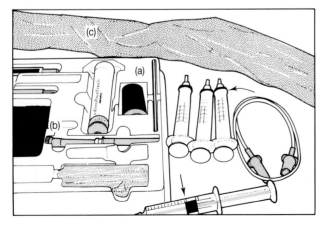

Fig. 7.1 A standard biopsy tray (A) for percutaneous biopsy with 10 ml syringes (curved arrow), syringe with local anaesthetic (arrow head), sterilizing solution (B) and transducer wrapped in sterile drape for protection (C).

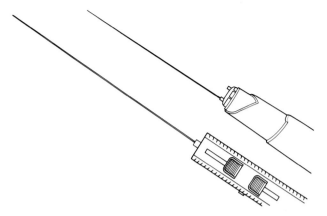

Fig. 7.3 Two examples of 18 gauge automated trigger devices that are disposable.

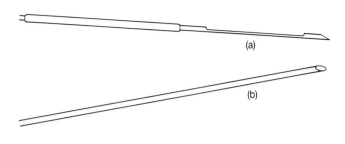

Fig. 7.4 (A) Close-up of an 18 gauge biopsy needle with a 17 mm core specimen clot exposed. (B) For positioning prior to biopsy, the inner needle is retracted into an outer sheath.

structed of disposable plastic or sterilizable metal (Fig. 7.3). They use an 18–20 gauge core needle with a 17 mm specimen notch at the distal aspect of its shaft (Fig. 7.4). Once triggered, the inner needle projects into the tissue and an outer cutting needle quickly glides over it leaving a specimen within the biopsy notch. The trauma and associated complications from these biopsies is very low. Even with the right equipment, an inability to locate the intended target will always defeat any biopsy attempt.

BIOPSY GUIDANCE

Originally, renal biopsies were performed blind, guided only by critical anatomical landmarks. This is no longer acceptable practice. All biopsy work should be guided by fluoroscopy, ultrasound (US) or computed tomography (CT). Ultrasound is the most dynamic and in the great majority of cases provides rapid and accurate localization.

Ultrasound

Sector scanners will have a pie-shaped image and linear scanners produce an image which is rectangular in shape. The sector-type probe has a small footprint reducing the overall size of the probe. The elements of a linear array transducer are arranged together in a series so the footprint is large. Both types are suitable, but the sector probe with its small footprint facilitates imaging between the ribs. In an

attempt to improve needle tip visualization with US, manufacturers have roughened the distal aspect of the shaft or placed crystals on the needle tip. This increases the number of acoustic interfaces available for interaction with the US beam. When the acoustic beam strikes a sono-view or sono-tipped needle, a focus of increased linear echoes will appear just proximal to the tip of the needle. The key to the success of US guidance is keeping the needle tip within a narrow sound field. This task is accomplished by using either a nonfixed (free hand) or a fixed (attachable needle guide) system.

The free-hand technique requires the use of both hands. One hand holds the transducer while the other guides the needle towards its designated target (Fig. 7.5). Because the needle is not confined within the enclosed space such as a plastic or metallic needle guide it is a nonrigid system. Once the needle enters the region of interest and is released, it can swing freely with the normal respiratory excursion which reduces the complication of a laceration injury to the kidney or adjacent structures.

The fixed system is rigid. Early models were designed so that the needle could pass through a hole within the transducer. Therefore, elements in the transducer foot plate had to be removed to allow access for the needle. Nonvisualization of the needle during its passage to the lesion became a major liability. As a fixed system, the chance of lacerating the kidney is increased. This complication is overcome by having biopsy guide attachments capable of quickly releasing the needle from its guide. Modern US guides attach to the side of a transducer and are plastic (disposable) or metallic (sterilizable and reusable) (Fig. 7.6). Each attachable guide has a preset angle which determines the angle of approach to the

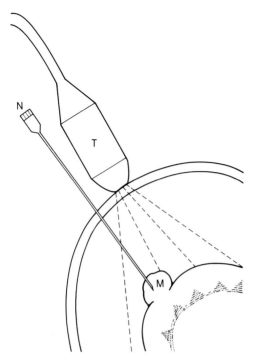

Fig. 7.5 Line drawing showing the free-hand method for guiding a 22 gauge Chiba needle (N) into a renal mass (M) with ultrasound.
T = transducer.

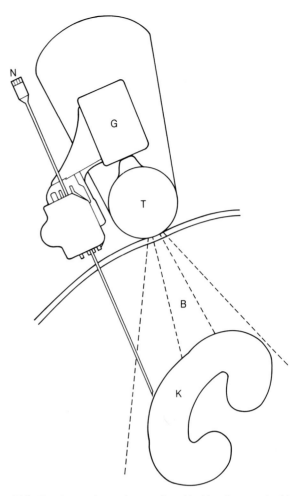

Fig. 7.6 This figure shows the needle guided by ultrasound with a guide (G) attached to the transducer (T). The needle (N) fits into a slot in the guide which has a fixed angle for guiding the needle into the sound beam (B) towards the kidney (K).

target (Fig. 7.7). The intended needle path is electronically projected onto the imaging screen and this ensures a more accurate localization. The polarity of the transducer must be considered when the guide is attached to the probe. If mismatching occurs, then the needle travels in a direction opposite to the one intended and visceral laceration will occur.

If the needle tip is not visualized with either the free-hand or the fixed technique, then some simple manoeuvres might help. The needle tip will not be seen in the first 1–2 cm of subcutaneous tissue.

1 Adjust the position of the transducer to redirect the beam to bring the needle tip into the image.
2 The inner stylet of the needle can be moved in a rapid up and down motion creating microbubbles at the needle tip. This act improves visualization by providing more surfaces to interact with the sound waves.
3 The needle tip itself can be oscillated up and down whilst continuous imaging and look for movement of the tissue surrounding the needle tip.

If these attempts fail, then the needle should be removed. Before its reinsertion, the needle path chosen and the polarity of the transducer should be checked. If a second attempt fails then a larger needle or a 'sonographically' tipped needle might be tried.

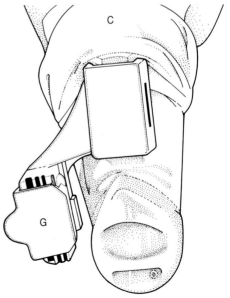

Fig. 7.7 (a) A sterile cover (C) is placed over the transducer and the attached guide (G) is presterilized.

Computed tomography

Computed tomography is needed where US fails. Patient habitus, a small fibrotic kidney blending with the adjacent perinephric fat, a lesion in an ectopic kidney or a very small lesion are the usual indications, although personal preference and experience may encourage some to perform most of their biopsies under CT guidance. Initial CT is performed to locate the lesion and a point on the skin directly above the lesion is marked, either with the aid of a metallic grid placed on the patient's skin or with the CT light beam. Registration difficulties often arise and it is important that the patient be encouraged to maintain the same phase of respiration for both scans and eventual biopsy. Once the site has been chosen, the patient is removed from the CT gantry, local anaesthesia is administered and the biopsy needle is inserted into the subcutaneous tissues. The patient is then repositioned within the gantry and an image acquired to check the position of the needle tip in the subcutaneous tissues relative to the lesion under investigation. The needle tip is then advanced in increments of 1–2 cm under intermittent CT control until it has reached the outer aspect of the lesion. The biopsy is then performed.

This is a time-consuming exercise, but is very accurate. One problem arises using core biopsy needles and an automatic triggering device. The device has to be mounted on the needle when it is advanced towards the lesion and removed from the needle during scanning. This can lead to the needle becoming displaced.

PATIENT SELECTION, PREPARATION AND POSITIONING

Relative contraindications to renal biopsy are:

1 A single functioning kidney
2 A bleeding diathesis
3 A small kidney (less than 8 cm)
5 Severe hypertension (diastolic pressure greater than 105 mm Hg).

Full informed consent and a clotting profile are needed. Urinary tract infections may contraindicate a renal biopsy for tissue diagnosis and appropriate antibiotics must be given. Bleeding and clotting times should be performed and if abnormal, cross-matching 1 or 2 units of blood is essential. If US

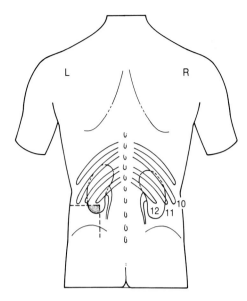

Fig. 7.8 Diagram of a patient in the prone position showing the optimum biopsy site at the outer inferior cortex of the lower pole (dotted line with shading).

guidance is planned, then a preprocedure scan will confirm that it is the appropriate modality and impending difficulties are anticipated.

Sampling renal masses for cytology can be performed on an outpatient basis, but core biopsy requires overnight observation in case haemorrhage complicates the biopsy. Further monitoring will vary with the type of biopsy done. If an intercostal approach is chosen, then post procedure inspiratory and expiratory chest films are needed to exclude a pneumothorax.

Most patients are positioned prone or prone–oblique for native renal biopsy (Fig. 7.8), but a supine approach is adopted for renal transplant biopsy or where the position of the target dictates (Fig. 7.9). To maintain the prone–oblique position, a bolster is placed under the side under investigation which has the net effect of elevating and fixing the kidney in a more horizontal orientation and separating the ribs improving access for a possible intercostal approach. When prone or prone–oblique, a biopsy needle should transverse only the retroperitoneal space reducing the chance of injury to visceral organs. An angled subcostal approach for the needle is desired with either position to avoid the lower margin of the pleura which can be as low as the ninth rib. With a vertical or intercostal approach, the risk of puncture of the pleural space resulting in a pneumothorax is increased.

Once the appropriate site is selected, it is marked by applying pressure to the skin surface using the hub of a needle. Waterproof ink is an alternative, but

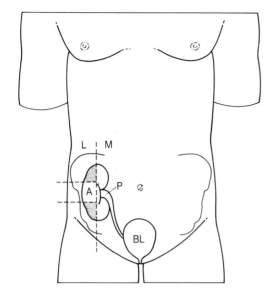

Fig. 7.9 Diagram of a renal transplant patient, supine, with the allograft positioned in the right iliac fossa.
Sites suitable for percutaneous biopsy (shaded) reside in the lower and upper poles. L = lateral kidney, M = medial kidney, A = allograft kidney. BL = bladder.

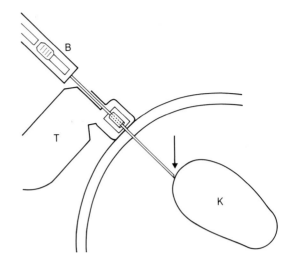

Fig. 7.10 Diagram showing the typical fixed guide system employed with ultrasound for directing an 18 gauge automated trigger needle (B) to the capsular margin of the native kidney (K). The tip of the needle only touches the capsule, but does not pass beyond (arrow). When triggered, the inner core needle will project through the capsule into cortex sampling the cortical glomeruli. T = transducer.

it may be erased when cleansing solutions are applied. Skin preparation begins with alcohol which removes the surface oils of the skin allowing deeper penetration of a topical sterilizing agent, for example, betadine. The skin and underlying soft tissues are infiltrated with a local anaesthetic agent and a small skin incision with a No.11 scalpel blade.

RENAL BIOPSY

The nephrologist will perform most renal biopsies with the radiologist providing assistance with localization and guidance. Indications for native kidney biopsy include:

1 Asymptomatic proteinuria
2 Microscopic haematuria
3 Idiopathic acute renal failure
4 Chronic renal impairment
5 Nephrotic syndrome.

A renal transplant biopsy is indicated when a structural abnormality is excluded as a reason for dysfunction.

For the native kidney, the lower poles of either kidney are biopsied. They are laterally and inferiorly situated away from the vascular pedicle. Biopsy is

usually performed with an automated trigger device and an 18 gauge needle. Best results are obtained by guiding the needle tip to the capsule of the kidney. Once the needle tip touches the capsule of the kidney, it is not advanced past it (Fig. 7.10). It is important to remember that the inner needle travels at least 2 cm and this distance must be taken into consideration. If the needle tip broaches the capsule first, then primarily medulla rather than cortex is sampled. At least two core specimens are usually obtained to ensure a sufficient amount of material is available for diagnostic studies.

Studies performed on these samples will vary depending on the needs of the nephrologist. The goal is to procure a sample with an adequate number of cortical glomeruli. Immediate examination of the specimen with a dissecting microscope helps in confirming the presence of cortical tissue and its glomeruli.

Nonvisualization of the needle tip is the primary pitfall of this procedure. The reasons for nonvisualization include:

1 Failure to match the polarity of the transducer with the side of the attached biopsy needle tip away from the intended target
2 Failure to select a path to the intended target properly

The fault does not generally lie with the gauge of the needle since an 18 gauge needle is well seen with US.

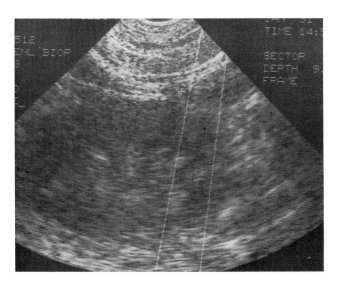

Fig. 7.11 A sagittal image of a native left kidney indicates the lower pole has been selected for biopsy. The double-dashed lines superimposed over the lower pole are guidance markers delineating the expected needle path.

If slight adjustments of the transducer do not bring the tip into sight, it is best to remove the needle completely and begin again. A careful re-evaluation will reveal one of the aforementioned problems (Fig 7.11). The upper and lower poles of renal transplants are biopsied. In general, a skin site slightly lateral to the position of the transplant is desired. This location reduces the likelihood of the needle entering the peritoneal cavity and transgressing bowel or other intra-abdominal organs. Particular attention should be given to the avoidance of the vascular pedicle, renal pelvis and ureter. Colour Doppler US is particularly useful in the transplant kidney allowing a path to be chosen which avoids any major intrarenal vessels.

Sometimes the capsule of the renal allograft becomes somewhat thickened from chronic inflammation. It may be so impervious to needle puncture that the needle deflects away from it. If this situation arises, then a sharp thrust onto the capsule may be required to achieve a suitable biopsy specimen.

COMPLICATIONS

Haemorrhage

Microscopic haematuria will occur in all cases. Macroscopic haematuria usually clears within 24h, but

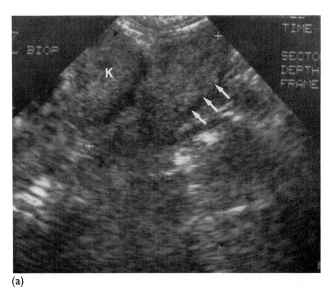

(a)

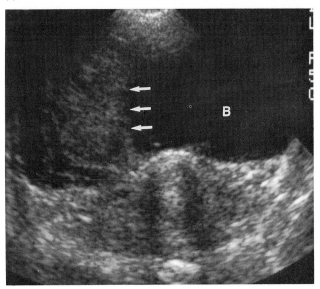

Fig. 7.12 (a) An amorphous collection of low level echoes are seen adjacent to the lower pole of a recently biopsied kidney (K). This moderate fixed haematoma (arrows) was easily seen on the postbiopsy ultrasound scan. (b) Transverse image of the bladder (B) with a collection of medium echoes along its right wall and also a haematoma (arrows).

may be severe enough to cause haemodynamic instability. Blood clot within the bladder may be large enough to cause urinary obstruction. Rarely, arteriovenous malformations or pseudoaneurysms may form. When small, they may regress spontaneously while larger ones usually require intervention (Fig. 7.12).

Haematoma

Haematomas frequently follow a biopsy of either the native or allograft kidney. These haematomas are usually small and of no consequence. When large, they can cause obstruction and renal vascular insufficiency due to a mass effect and may require percutaneous drainage.

BIOPSY OF RENAL MASSES

Renal mass aspiration or biopsy is reserved for cases where distinction between a benign and malignant lesion is in doubt and to differentiate between a primary renal malignancy and a metastasis. Biopsy is not indicated when surgery is planned irrespective of the biopsy outcome. This is because of potential seeding of the needle track by neoplasm following a large core biopsy, especially cystic papillary renal cell carcinoma. Success of renal mass aspiration and biopsy begins with careful pre-biopsy assessment and planning. All prior imaging studies are scrutinized so that the exact location, vascularity, consistency and extent of the lesion are known. From this information, the best needle approach, needle type and guidance modality will be chosen. Although US is preferred, CT guidance is often employed when a lesion is small and difficult to image with US and when it is important to biopsy the wall of a lesion.

In most cases, adequate cytologic specimens are obtained with needles ranging between 22 and 23 gauge, for example, Chiba, spinal, Menghini and Turner needles. Manufacturers have made available similar needles with a 'sono-tip' to enhance US visualization. More rarely a core specimen may be needed, but if it is, a 20 gauge biopsy needle with an automatic trigger device is used. Biopsy is performed with the patient in suspended respiration. Once the mass has been entered, the needle is released and the patient is allowed to breath shallowly. If the patient breaths with the needle fixed, it may be dislodged from the mass or lacerate the kidney. Aspiration of the mass begins with the removal of the inner stylet of the needle and attaching a 5–10 ml locking syringe to the hub of the needle. Then, the plunger is pulled back to provide suction and the needle-syringe unit moved rapidly up and down three to five times over a 1 to 2 cm distance to obtain tissue. As the needle is withdrawn from the mass, suction is released on the syringe. The whole process must be completed within seconds since the patient

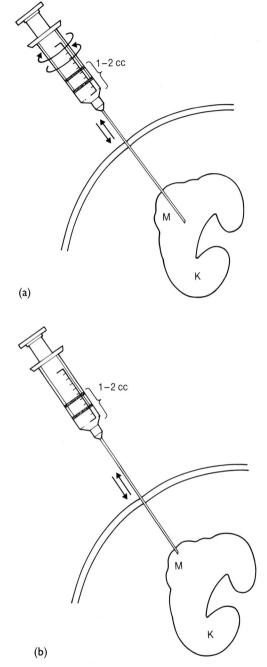

(a)

(b)

Fig. 7.13 Diagram showing a 10 ml syringe attached to a 22 gauge needle which has been inserted into a renal mass.
The arrows indicate the up/down motion required for aspiration for cytological material. K = kidney. M = mass.

is encourage to suspend respiration during the process of sampling. This procedure is repeated three to five times ensuring adequate sampling (Fig. 7.13a and b).

To obtain core specimens, a cutting type needle or a larger needle such as an 18 or 20 gauge needle is needed. Sterile saline, 1 to 2 ml, is added to the syringe and a circular clockwise and counterclockwise rotation is made in conjunction with the up and down motion of the syringe–needle unit. This manoeuvre frees a large proportion of tissue needed for the core specimen.

False-positive and false-negative results are reduced by having a skilled cytologist present to review each sample. Even though a sample is deemed adequate on the first pass, a second sampling should be performed to avoid a sampling error. When the cytologist is unavailable, samples are placed in formalin or other medium for immediate transport to the laboratory.

Several pitfalls may be encountered leading to insufficient specimens. Commonly, a fine needle will bend or deflect from its intended target. It lacks the stiffness demanded for the distance to be travelled by it. As a remedy, a larger, 18 gauge needle may be directed through the retroperitoneal soft tissues, but short of the kidney mass. Its inner stylet is replaced by the 22 gauge fine needle. The protected inner fine needle is advanced through the sturdier 18 gauge needle. Now, the unprotected portion of the fine needle travels a short distance to the mass. Other common mistakes include failure to consider transducer polarity, misapplication of the guide to the transducer and failure to consider depth.

Occasionally, the internal consistency of a mass will contribute to the acquisition of an insufficient specimen. In this case, the mass is usually large with central necrosis. A sample from this inner portion usually contains necrotic debris and too few viable cells for a specific cytologic diagnosis. This pitfall is averted by sampling the peripheral segment where many viable cells reside (Fig. 7.14).

A mass in the upper pole region of the kidney should be approached with caution because it may be extrarenal in origin. The unsuspected pheochromocytoma is worrisome since manipulation of it can lead to a severe, hypertensive crisis. To exclude this entity, a 24 h urinary vanillylmandelic acid (VMA) or urinary catecholamine level should be determined. Otherwise, one must be prepared to manage a hypertensive crisis during the biopsy.

Rarely has neoplastic seeding of the biopsy tract has been documented and it remains an infrequent complication. To reduce this risk, some investigators have advocated instillation of 1 to 2 ml sterile water into the site prior to withdrawal of the needle. This procedure should lyse the few neoplastic cells that spill into the tract after biopsy.

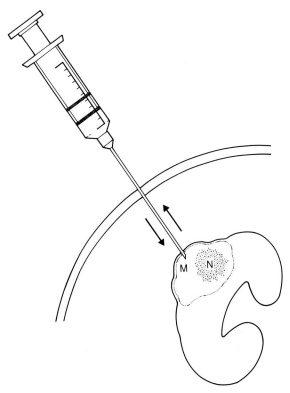

Fig. 7.14 Diagram showing the technique for biopsy of the peripheral portion of a necrotic renal mass. Notice the needle tip is in the solid tissue at the periphery of the lesion away from the necrotic central part. N = necrotic centre. M = mass.

SUGGESTED FURTHER READING

BEAMAN M (1969) How to perform a renal biopsy. *British Journal of Hospital Medicine* **41**: 158–60.

BUSH WH Jr, BURNETT LL, GIBONS RP (1977) Needle tract seeding of renal cell carcinoma. *American Journal of Radiology* **129**: 595–6.

HURAID S, GOLDBERG H, KATZ A *et al.* (1989) Percutaneous needle biopsy of the transplant kidney: echnique and complications. *American Journal of Kidney Diseases* 13–14.

LINDSAY DJ, LYONS EA, LEVI CS (1990) Urinary tract. In: *Interventional Ultrasound*, pp. 199–210. Edited by McGahan JP. Williams and Wilkins, Baltimore.

ROWLEY VA, COOPERBERG PL (1987) Ultrasound guided biopsy. In: *Interventional Ultrasound Clinics in Diagnostic Ultrasound*, pp. 59–76. Edited by Van Sonnenberg E. Churchill Livingstone, New York.

WEHLE MJ, GRABSTALD H (1986) Contraindications to needle aspiration of a solid renal mass: tumour dissemination by renal needle aspiration. *Journal of Urology* **136**: 446–8.

CHAPTER 8

Percutaneous drainage of renal and perirenal fluid collections

Rick Feld, Joseph Bonn and Matthew D. Rifkin

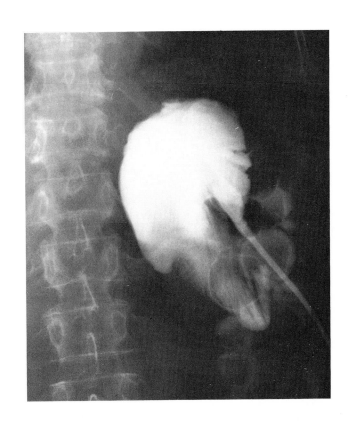

INTRODUCTION

Percutaneous drainage of abdominal and retroperitoneal fluid collections has become a widely accepted means of nonsurgical therapy. Recent series have shown reduced morbidity and mortality of percutaneous catheter therapy versus surgical drainage. The most common fluid collections related to the kidney are abscess, haematoma, uriniferous collections and lymphocoele. Although both computed tomography (CT) and ultrasound (US) image retroperitoneal collection, contrast-enhanced CT is preferable as the initial study since daughter abscesses, areas of loculations, gas within the collection and the full extent of the collection are more evident. Ultrasound has the advantage of being portable allowing bedside evaluation in the critically ill patient.

ANATOMY

The relationship of the kidney to the fascial layers of the retroperitoneum is vital to understanding the origin and spread of fluid collections (Fig. 8.1). The renal parenchyma is surrounded by a fibrous capsule. The perirenal space contains the kidney, surrounding fat and the adrenal gland. This space is closed superiorly and laterally but may communicate inferiorly with the anterior and posterior pararenal spaces and across the midline to the contralateral perirenal space. Almost all collections in this space are renal in origin including abscess extension, haemorrhage and neoplasm. Extensive pancreatic processes may also involve the perirenal space. The anterior pararenal space is delineated by the posterior peritoneum of the abdominal cavity and the anterior renal fascia. The lateroconal fascia forms its lateral boundary. This space contains the pancreas, duodenum, fat, and ascending and descending colon. Fluid collections derived from the pancreas (abscess and pseudocyst) as well as abscess formation related to bowel (retroceacal appendicitis, diverticulitis and duodenal trauma) will localize in this space. The posterior pararenal space is located between the posterior renal fascia and transversalis fascia. This space contains fat, but no organs and communicates in the pelvis with the anterior pararenal space.

The flank approach provides the best extraperitoneal access route to most renal fluid collections. It is important to realize that retrorenal extension of the peritoneal cavity may occur. It is

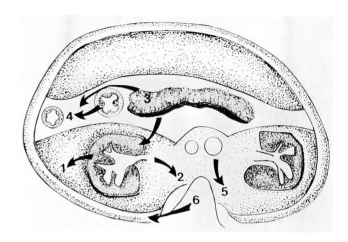

Fig. 8.1 Diagram illustrating the common routes of spread of retroperitoneal fluid collections.
(1) Renal abscess with extension to the perinephric space. (2) Urinoma with extension to the perinephric space. (3) Pancreatic fluid collections with extension to either the anterior pararenal space or perinephric space. (4) Gastrointestinal perforation with extension to the anterior pararenal space. (5) Leaking abdominal aortic aneurysm with extension to the perinephric space. (6) Osteomyelitis of the spine with extension to the posterior pararenal space. Modified with permission from Davidson, Alan, *Radiology of the Kidney*, W. B. Saunders, 1985, p. 630.

therefore possible that loops of small bowel, ascites and solid organs including the liver and spleen may be interposed between the flank and a potential collection. This anatomic variation is relevant to catheter drainage.

CLINICAL CONSIDERATIONS

Abscess

Abscesses are frequently insidious in presentation and the clinical diagnosis is often difficult. Most renal, perirenal and pararenal fluid collections present with a history of flank pain or fever. Factors predisposing to abscess include diabetes mellitus, obstructive uropathy, renal calculi, polycystic kidney disease, paraplegia, alcoholism, recent surgery and immunodeficiency such as in renal transplantation. Perinephric abscess occurs more commonly in the elderly. Urine cultures reflect the causative organism in 70% of cases, the most common being *Escherichia coli, Proteus mirabilis,* enteric Gram negatives such as *Klebsiella pneumoniae* and *Pseudomonas aeruginosa.*

Percutaneous diagnostic aspiration is indicated when a complex fluid collection is identified in the

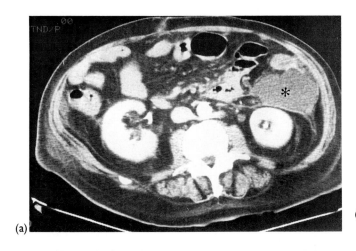

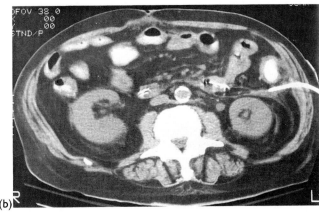

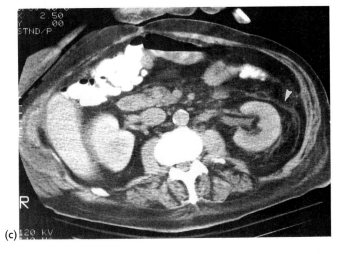

Fig. 8.2 Computed tomography (a) demonstrating a large fluid collection (*) in the anterior pararenal space. (b) following catheter drainage, and (c) at 3 months showing residual post-infective thickening of the renal fascia.

clinical setting of an abscess. The decision regarding catheter placement depends upon the size and location of the collection, the nature of the diagnostic aspirate and the presence of a safe access route. Computed tomography is useful to localize a collection to the renal, perirenal or pararenal spaces, especially if the abscess has gas within it, a feature which degrades US images. Ultrasound characterizes the fluid better, demonstrating septations, internal echoes and fluid debris levels. A small abscess (< 2 cm) localized within the renal capsule may be effectively treated by complete needle aspiration. When renal calculi are associated with abscess, colonization on the surface of the stone tends to render appropriate antibiotics ineffective. Drainage as well as percutaneous or surgical stone removal is needed.

Large purulent collections require catheter drainage (Fig. 8.2). Original criteria for percutaneous abscess drainage of abdominal collections (renal and nonrenal) were limited to unilocular, well-defined collections. For this group of patients, catheter drainage may be used as a temporizing measure prior to definitive surgery. Most perirenal abscesses orig-

inate within the renal parenchyma and rupture through the renal fascia to involve the perirenal space. Perirenal abscess tends to be lobular in configuration and extend along the facial plane to assume an elongated shape along the psoas muscle.

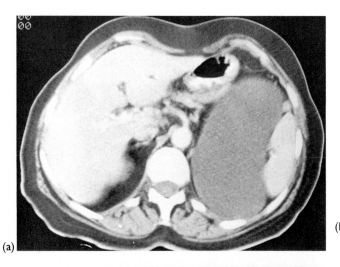

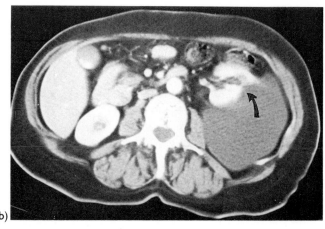

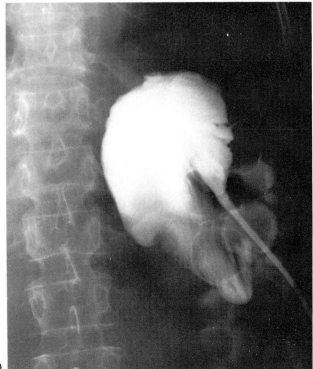

Fig. 8.3 (a) Computed tomography shows a large fluid collection compressing the spleen, (b) same collection related to a middle pole calyx (arrow). (c) Sinogram following catheter drainage demonstrating communication of the fluid collection with the pelvicalyceal system.

fibrous tissue forming a pseudocyst usually situated inferomedial to the lower pole of the kidney and displacing the proximal ureter medially. The clinical presentation may include a palpable flank mass and vague abdominal tenderness occurring over months. Significant fever is uncommon. Urine may also leak into the perinephric space secondary to acute obstruction or trauma and this collection will not be encapsulated (Fig. 8.3 a–c). In acute obstruction, elevation of hydrostatic pressure in the pelvicalyceal system causes rupture of a calyceal fornix. Percutaneous catheter management includes both drainage of the uriniferous collection as well as percutaneous nephrostomy or antegrade stent placement to relieve hydronephrosis or urine leak (Fig. 8.4 a–e). The level and perhaps aetiology of the obstruction can then be defined.

Uriniferous collections

Urinoma is a chronic collection of urine localized outside the renal collecting system, ureter or urinary bladder. Leakage of urine into the perinephric space may occur secondary to a disruption in the collecting system or proximal ureter especially with chronic ureteral obstruction. The most common causes are chronic distal obstruction secondary to ureteral stone, neoplasm or periureteric fibrosis. With time, the urine collection becomes encapsulated by fatty-

Haematoma

Perinephric haematoma occurs with blunt or penetrating abdominal trauma (including percutaneous needle biopsy), a leaking abdominal aortic aneurysm, haemorrhage from a retroperitoneal tumour (e.g. renal cell carcinoma, hamartoma, metastasis and simple cyst), renal infarction or secondary to an underlying bleeding diathesis. These patients

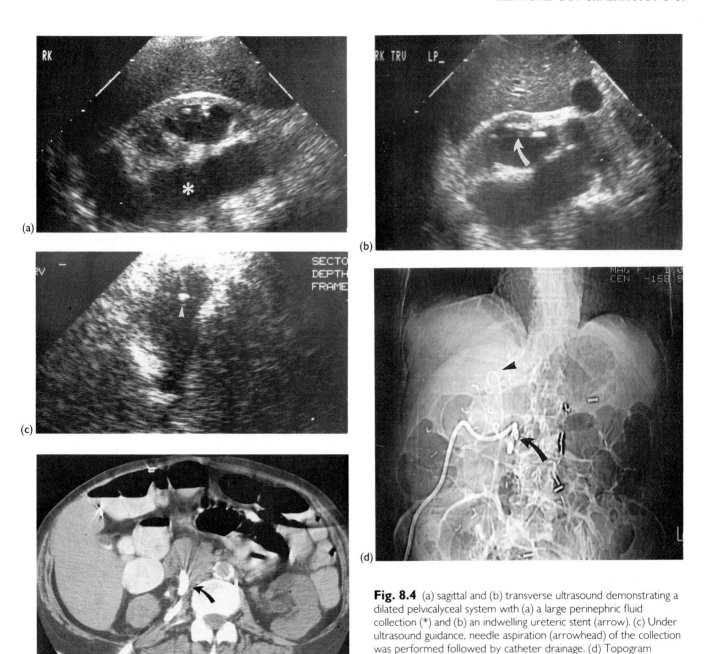

Fig. 8.4 (a) sagittal and (b) transverse ultrasound demonstrating a dilated pelvicalyceal system with (a) a large perinephric fluid collection (*) and (b) an indwelling ureteric stent (arrow). (c) Under ultrasound guidance, needle aspiration (arrowhead) of the collection was performed followed by catheter drainage. (d) Topogram demonstrating a pigtail drainage catheter (arrow) and the double 'J' stent (arrowhead). (e) Computed tomography following 1 month's drainage showing the catheter in the paraspinal collection.

may have mild fever. Most subcapsular haematomas will extend into the perirenal space. Acute haemorrhage is equal to or greater in attenuation than renal cortex on CT. With time, the collection will haemolyse and attenuation values decrease within 1 month. Haematomas usually resolve spontaneously and catheter drainage is indicated only to relieve mass effect or when percutaneous aspiration demonstrates evidence of infection either by Gram stain or culture.

Lymphocoele

Lymphocoele is most commonly due to surgical disruption of lymphatic vascular channels. Following pelvic lymphadenectomy, lymph may accumulate in the operative site, resulting in an encysted lymphatic fluid collection. These collections usually occur within 2 months of surgery. They can produce obstructive uropathy by pressure effects on the distal ureter.

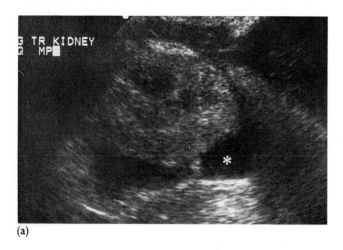

(a)

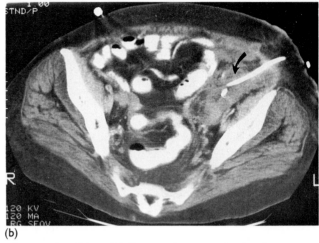

(b)

Fig. 8.5 (a) Ultrasound demonstraing a complex fluid collection (*) around a transplant kidney. (b) Computed tomography showing a draining catheter within the collection avoiding bowel loops (arrow).

RENAL TRANSPLANT COLLECTIONS

Renal transplantation is an accepted means of therapy in patients with end stage renal disease. Peritransplant fluid collections are identified in as many as 50% of cases. Lymphocoeles are the most common and are located medial or inferior to the lower pole of the transplant. They are commonly associated with hydronephroses and diminished graft function. Urinomas are also frequently detected in the early postoperative period, usually 1–2 weeks post-transplantation, resulting from leakage from the renal pelvis, ureteroneocystostomy or urinary bladder. They are usually located near the lower pole of the transplant or near the bladder. Treatment of urinoma should include percutaneous nephrostomy drainage and stenting, if any leaks are demonstrated. Abscess generally occurs 5–6 weeks following surgery with a variable location (Fig. 8.5a and b). Haematoma is less common than other fluid collections and also tends to occur late. Ultrasound offers the best imaging modality. The appearances are nonspecific. Septations are more common in lymphocoele and haematoma, but may be seen in abscess; they are rarely seen in urinoma. Percutaneous aspiration or drainage is indicated for the treatment of abscess and for the relief of mass effect (e.g. hydronephroses secondary to lymphocoele). Lymphocoeles often recur and may require surgical drainage.

The most common surgical site for renal transplantation is in either iliac fossa which allows vascular anastomoses to the iliac arteries and vein. The transplant is retroperitoneal in location. The safest access route for a perirenal transplant collection is as lateral as possible to avoid loops of bowel and more medially situated vascular anastomoses. The axis of the transplant kidney is medially rotated and the vascular anastomosis is usually an end-to-side renal artery to external iliac artery and end-to-side renal vein to external iliac vein. With multiple renal arteries in the donor kidney, a patch of aorta may be used to the side of the external iliac artery. Urinary drainage is commonly performed by uretero neocystostomy. Unless planning a percutaneous nephrostomy drainage, traversing the transplant kidney by either a diagnostic aspiration needle or drainage catheter should be avoided.

TECHNIQUE OF CATHETER DRAINAGE

Informed consent and a clotting profile should be obtained. If infection or an abscess is suspected, broad-spectrum antibiotics with a dosage according to renal function should be administered.

As with any interventional radiological procedure, review of all prior imaging studies is essential. Absolute contraindications to percutaneous drainage are an uncorrectable coagulopathy and lack of a safe access route. Relative contraindications are the presence of multiple abscesses, microabscesses and necrotic, infected neoplasm. Contrast-enhanced

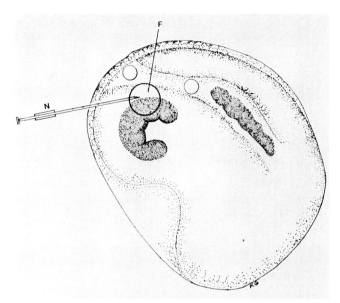

Fig. 8.6 Diagram illustrating that the most direct access to a perinephric fluid collection is achieved with the patient in either an anterior oblique (shown) or prone position. Modified with permission from Meyers, Morton A., *Dynamic Radiology of the Abdomen*, Springer Verlag, 1976, p. 118.
F=fluid, N=aspirating needle.

CT will best be able to help plan the route of access to a fluid collection that is free of bowel, vascular structures and pleural reflections. Although fine needles (20 gauge or less) may traverse the bowel with safety, a pathway free of the bowel even for the diagnostic aspiration is best to avoid confusing Gram stain and culture results secondary to bowel contamination. The optimal drainage route should be as direct as possible using an extraperitoneal approach. Renal fluid collections are best drained through the posterior flank, right posterior oblique for the left kidney and left posterior oblique for the right kidney (Fig. 8.6)

To be certain that a catheter will not traverse the pleural space, one should stay below the 12th rib if possible, but definitely below the 10th rib. To avoid colon, obviously correlate with the CT scan, but remain posterior to the midaxillary line.

For the initial diagnostic aspiration, a 20 gauge spinal or Chiba needle is preferred. It is small enough to allow aspiration of almost all fluid collections, except the most viscous. The aspirate from an abscess is cloudy, purulent and usually free flowing. Aspirate from a haematoma is usually serosanguinous and characteristically yields only a small amount of material (1–2 ml), being rather difficult and tenacious to aspirate. Uriniferous collections will look (and smell) like urine and are clear yellow; a creatinine concentration measured from this specimen will be greater than serum creatinine and confirm its origin. Lymphocoele fluid is clear or straw coloured. Biochemical tests on the aspirate are only necessary if the diagnosis is not apparent from the gross appearance (Table 8.1). A specimen must be sent from any aspirate for microbiology tests including aerobic and anaerobic cultures as well as fungal cultures for immunosuppressed patients. A gram stain is useful if there is doubt. The presence of organisms and numerous white cells indicates the necessity for catheter drainage. If organisms and only a few white blood cells are identified, the aspiration may have originated from the colon. If absolutely no fluid can be obtained then aspiration with an 18 gauge needle should be performed.

Sterile technique is employed. Local anaesthesia for diagnostic aspiration and intravenous analgesia for catheter insertion is normally used. Supplemental nasal cannula oxygen may be necessary.

A catheter can be placed within the collection by one or two methods, either the Seldinger technique (Fig. 8.7) or the tandem trochar technique (Fig. 8.8). There are advantages and disadvantages to each approach. The Seldinger technique employs serial dilations by fascial dilators placed over an indwelling (0.038 inch) guidewire. The catheter is then placed and the guidewire is removed. This technique allows more precise control over the catheter and although it is more time consuming, it is preferred for deep and small collections. The tandem trochar technique utilizes the path of the initial diagnostic puncture needle, which is left in place. The tandem trochar

	Appearance	Viscosity	Biochemistry
Abscess	Cloudy Creamy	Free flowing but may be more viscous	Exudate
Haematoma	Serosanguinous and difficult to aspirate	Extremely viscous	Exudate
Uriniferous	Clear yellow	Free flowing	Transudate, creatinine>serum
Lymphocoele	Clear or coloured	Free flowing	Exudate, creatinine<serum

Table 8.1 *Gross and biochemical characteristics of an aspirate*

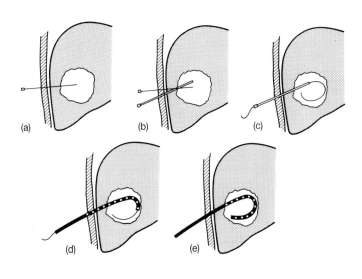

Fig. 8.7 Diagram illustrating the Seldinger technique for abscess drainage.
(a) Ultrasound or computed tomographic guided diagnostic aspiration (20 gauge Chiba or spinal needle). (b) Tandem puncture with a larger cannula or 18 gauge needle; aspiration should yield fluid or purulent material. (c) Under fluoroscopic control, an 0.038 inch guidewire is advanced into the cavity followed by removal of the needle and serial fascial dilators over the guidewire. (d) Large bore multi-side hole catheter is introduced over the guidewire and positioned so that it is situated at the most dependent portion of the cavity with all the side holes within the cavity. (e) The guidewire is withdrawn and all accessible fluid is aspirated and drained.
Reprinted with permission from Ferrucci, Joseph T, et al., *Interventional Radiology of the Abdomen*, Williams and Wilkins, 1985, p. 125.

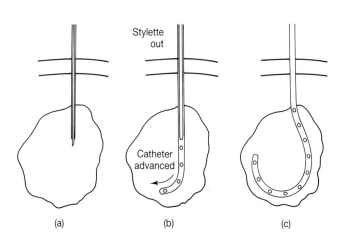

Fig. 8.8 Diagram illustrating the tandem trochar technique for abscess drainage.
(a) Catheter/cannula/trochar stylet are advanced as a locked unit in tandem fashion under ultrasound or computed tomography guidance. (b) Catheter is advanced into the dependent portion of the cavity while the stiffening cannula is held stationary. (c) Stiffening cannula is removed and catheter fixed in place by a molnar disc or stoma device. Complete aspiration is performed.
Reprinted with permission from Ferrucci, Joseph T. et al., *Interventional Radiology of the Abdomen*, Williams and Wilkins, 1985, p. 133.

consists of an inner stylet, stiff cannula and overlying catheter which is advanced alongside the diagnostic needle in the cavity. It is important to use a definitive deep scalpel incision into the subcutaneous tissue followed by widening of the tract with a haemostat to facilitate passage of the trocar. The inner trocar stylet is removed and aspiration of fluid at this point confirms the position of the tip in the cavity. The overlying catheter is subsequently advanced over the stiffening cannula which is held stationary. The trochar technique is advisable only for large and superficial collections where there is no question of jeopardizing adjacent bowel. It is performed more rapidly than the Seldinger technique but may cause more patient discomfort during insertion.

The drainage catheter may occasionally telescope or collapse during insertion by either the Seldinger or tandem trocar technique and not pass easily over the guidewire or stiffening cannula. In such a case, larger fascial dilators over a stiffer guidewire are

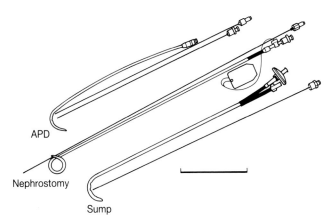

APD

Nephrostomy

Sump

Fig. 8.9 Commercially available catheters for drainage of fluid collections include the all-purpose drainage (APD) catheter, pigtail nephrostomy catheter and Van Sonnenberg sump, each with an inner stylet and stiffening cannula.

necessary prior to catheter insertion.

A wide variety of drainage catheters with multiple sideholes are commercially available (Fig. 8.9). The all purpose drainage (APD) catheter (Meditech, Watertown, MA, USA) has a gentle curve at its distal end. The Cope loop catheter (Cook Urological, Spencer, IN, USA) has the advantage of a locking loop at the distal end. The nephrostomy pigtail catheter (Meditech, Watertown, MA, USA) has a self-retaining loop at the distal end. The Van Sonnenberg sump catheter (Meditech, Watertown, MA, USA), for the largest collections, has a double lumen, the larger of which allows fluid egress drainage while the smaller lumen allows ingress of filtered air to allow continuous suction and has a gentle curve at its distal end. Catheter sizes range from 8 Fr to 14 Fr.

Depending on the technology available in a given institution, drainage may be performed with a combination of either US, CT or fluoroscopy. A large superficial collection could be aspirated and drained by the trocar technique entirely in either the CT or US suite. A portable US unit could be brought to the fluoroscopy suite where diagnostic aspiration performed under US guidance would allow passage of a guidewire. Fluoroscopy could then be utilized for the passage of dilators and catheter by the Seldinger technique. Alternatively, a guidewire can be positioned in a cavity under CT guidance. The patient would then be transported to the fluoroscopy suite for definitive catheter placement by the Seldinger technique. The most important therapeutic effect of percutaneous abscess drainage occurs at initial drainage; aspiration of as much purulent material as possible should be performed. If the material becomes sanguineous, or ceases to flow easily, aspiration should be discontinued. Following evacuation

of the cavity, opinions vary regarding irrigation of the cavity; this may be performed gently with sterile saline, although there is a risk of provoking bacteraemia and septic shock.

The catheter is left to gravity drainage via an extension tube with orders for strict recordings of outputs by nursing staff. The catheter should be flushed once a day with a small amount (5–10 ml) of sterile saline. For abscess, clinical response to drainage is the most important indicator of success and the fever curve and leucocyte count should be closely monitored. For urinoma, lymphocele and hematoma, fluid output from the catheter should be closely followed. Catheters should be checked and repositioned under fluoroscopy as necessary. Once drainage falls below 10 ml/day, the catheter may be clamped. If a follow-up CT or fluoroscopic sinogram 48 hours later demonstrates no evidence of reaccumulation the catheter may be removed. A Cope loop or pigtail nephrostomy catheter should be removed only over a stiff guidewire such as an Amplatz wire.

SUGGESTED FURTHER READING

BERNARDINO, ME and BAUMGARTNER BR (1986) Abscess drainage in the genitourinary tract. *Radiologic Clinics of North America* **24**: 539–49.

DAVIDSON, AJ (1985) The retroperitoneum. In: *Radiology of the Kidney*, pp. 640–5. W.B. Saunders, Philadelphia.

FERRUCCI, JT and MUELLER, PR (1985) Catheter drainage of abdominal abscesses and fluid collection: indications, technique, and instrumentation. In: *Interventional Radiology of the Abdomen*, pp. 8 108–44. Edited by Ferrucci JT, Wittenberg J, Mueller PR, and Simeone JF. Williams and Wilkins, Baltimore.

HANTO, DW and SIMMONS, RL (1987) Renal transplantion: Clinical considerations. *Radiologic Clinics of North America* **25**: 239–48.

LANG EK and GLORIOSO L (1986) Management of urinomas by percutaneous drainage procedures. *Radiologic Clinics of North America* **24**: 551–59.

LANG EK (1990) Renal, perirenal, and pararenal abscesses: percutaneous drainage. *Radiology* **174**: 109–13.

PATTERSON JE and ANDRIOLE VT (1987) Renal and perirenal abscesses. *Infectious Disease Clinics of North America* **1**: 907–26.

VANSONNENBERG E, MUELLER PR and FERRUCCI JT (1984) Percutaneous drainage of 250 abdominal abscesses and fluid collections. *Radiology* **150**: 337–41.

YODER IC and PFISTER RC (1990) Drainage of abscesses and fluid collections. In: *Clinical Urography*, pp. 2818–27. Edited by Pollack HM, WB Saunders, Philadelphia.

Diagnostic urogenital arteriography

Neale A. Walters and Ken R. Thomson

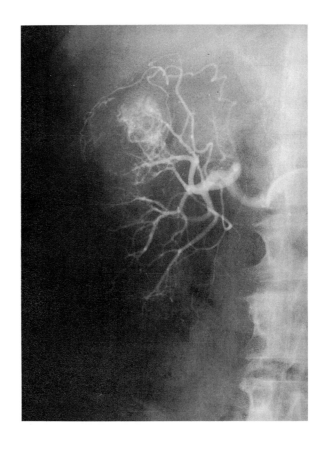

PATIENT PREPARATION

Prior to angiography, informed consent must be obtained from adult patients. The radiologist must be aware of the indications for the study which always requires consultation with the referring clinician. The patient's diagnosis may be made by less invasive techniques such as magnetic resonance imaging (MRI) or computed tomography (CT), but it is not cost-effective to perform alternative tests when the angiogram will be required whatever the outcome of other tests.

All normal medications should be taken as usual with free oral fluids. A light meal may be taken before the procedure. Hungry patients are less cooperative and swallow gas which interferes with digital subtraction examinations. If the patient has extensive abdominal gas, then intravenous Buscopan or glucagon may be given to stop gas misregistration when digital subtraction angiography (DSA) is being used. Routine premedication is not recommended. The majority of patients respond well to a confident team of people performing the examination and being given the opportunity to talk about the procedure. Anxious patients should be premedicated with oral diazepam 2 hours before the procedure or an intravenous dose immediately before it starts. General anaesthesia is reserved for confused patients, children and when a phaeochromocytoma is suspected. Such patients need α- and β-adrenergic blockade with popranolol and phentolamine prior to the procedure which should be performed under general anaesthesia.

The patient must be continuously monitored. The Dinamap monitor (Model 845, Critikon Inc 1982, Tampa, Florida 33622) is ideal and unobtrusive.

CONTRAST MEDIA

The risks of diagnostic arteriography are low and complications are infrequent. In our laboratory, complications are less than 0.5%. Low osmolar nonionic contrast medium is exclusively used. Although the toxicity of iodinated media has improved dramatically with respect to idiosyncratic reactions, there is still a risk of a temporary reduction in renal function which is more probable if the patient is dehydrated, elderly or receives a large dose of contrast medium selectively into one or both renal arteries.

Embolization with cholesterol from diseased vessels may be the cause of some cases of 'contrast medium-induced' renal failure as seen on renal biopsy in affected patients. Cholesterol embolization is certainly more likely to occur following angioplasty than simple diagnostic procedures.

PROCEDURAL COMPLICATIONS

Dissection of an artery by a catheter or guidewire is more probable when a superselective catheter is placed into the renal artery or when it is narrowed due to arteriosclerosis. Catheterization of a severe stenosis using a deflecting wire or with a stiff Simmons shaped catheter may also result in dissection. Spasm produced by a superselective catheter is common and may cause the procedure to be aborted. Small dissections or spasm only rarely cause symptoms or lasting complications.

Bleeding at the puncture site is more likely if the patient is very hypertensive (systolic pressure over 180 mm Hg), if the patient is obese or if the artery is heavily calcified at the puncture site. The size of the catheter used is less important than the weight of the patient in the incidence of haematoma formation after arteriography. The major cause of severe hypertension before angiography is failure of the patient to take antihypertensive medication because they were told to fast for 12 hours before the procedure.

If during the procedure the patient experiences flank pain, it should immediately be reported to the radiologist. During angioplasty, some discomfort is usual as the balloon is inflated to its maximum diameter, but the discomfort should end as the balloon is deflated. If the pain persists, this may indicate ischaemia of a portion of the kidney or rupture of the renal artery. If flank pain occurs during diagnostic angiography, then it may indicate contrast extravasation, dissection of the artery or severe spasm produced by the catheter. The authors use an 'operation sheet' upon which the procedure and monitoring can be recorded (Fig. 9.1). This is essential for interventional procedures which should be documented with the same care as conventional surgery.

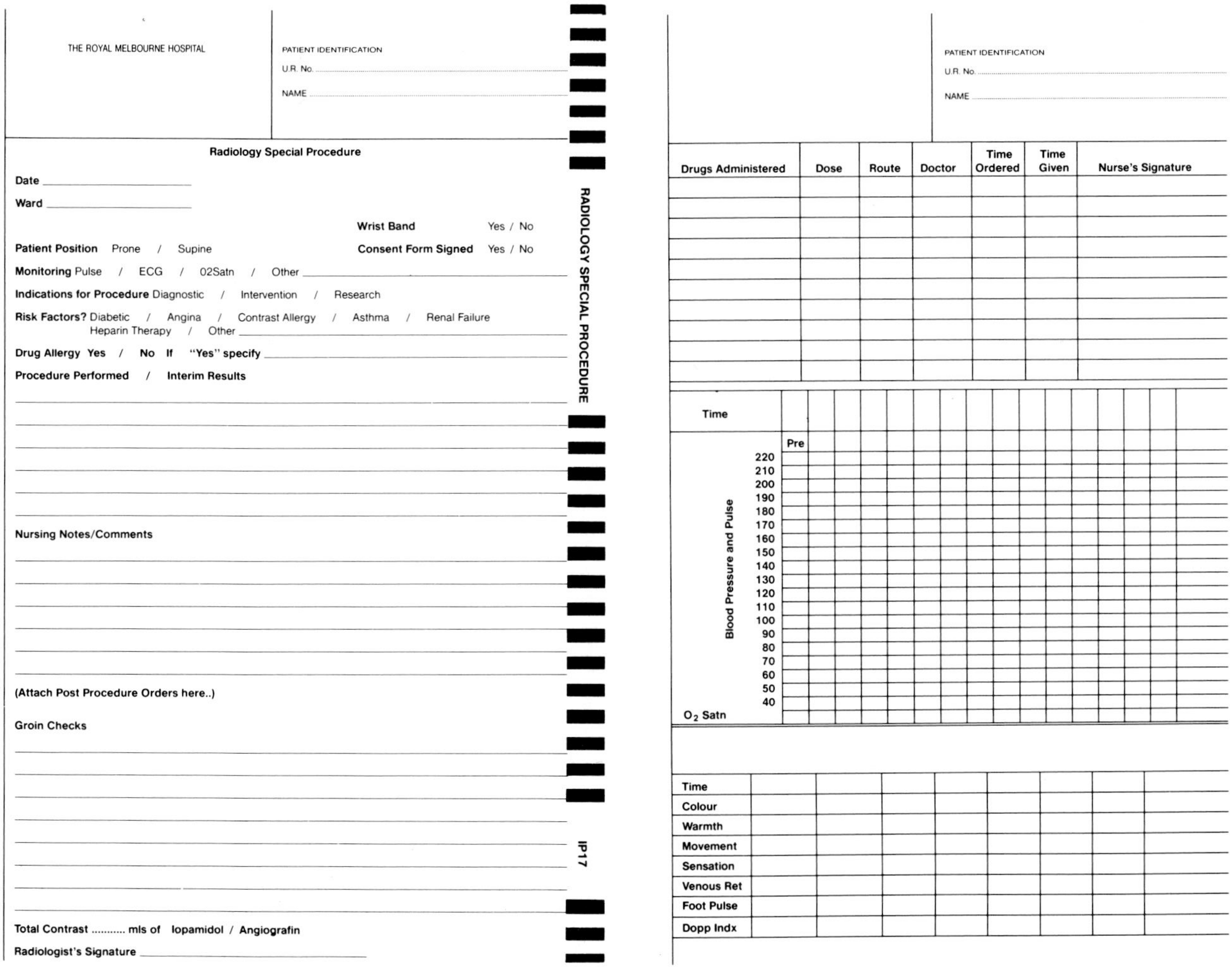

THE ROYAL MELBOURNE HOSPITAL

PATIENT IDENTIFICATION

U.R. No. _____

NAME _____

RADIOLOGY SPECIAL PROCEDURE

Radiology Special Procedure

Date _____

Ward _____

Wrist Band   Yes / No

Patient Position   Prone / Supine   Consent Form Signed   Yes / No

Monitoring Pulse / ECG / 02Satn / Other _____

Indications for Procedure Diagnostic / Intervention / Research

Risk Factors? Diabetic / Angina / Contrast Allergy / Asthma / Renal Failure
Heparin Therapy / Other _____

Drug Allergy Yes / No   If   "Yes" specify _____

Procedure Performed / Interim Results

_____
_____
_____
_____

Nursing Notes/Comments

_____
_____
_____
_____

(Attach Post Procedure Orders here..)

Groin Checks

_____
_____
_____
_____

Total Contrast .... mls of   Iopamidol / Angiografin

Radiologist's Signature _____

PATIENT IDENTIFICATION

U.R. No. _____

NAME _____

Drugs Administered	Dose	Route	Doctor	Time Ordered	Time Given	Nurse's Signature

Time

Blood Pressure and Pulse

Pre
220
210
200
190
180
170
160
150
140
130
120
110
100
90
80
70
60
50
40

O₂ Satn

Time					
Colour					
Warmth					
Movement					
Sensation					
Venous Ret					
Foot Pulse					
Dopp Indx					

IP17

Fig. 9.1 Operation sheet for arteriographic and interventional procedures. This is modelled on an operation report and is a complete record of the procedure itself.

EQUIPMENT OPTIONS

A high-quality fluoroscope and film acquisition system is essential. The capability to perform magnification conventional films as well as DSA is desirable, but perfectly adequate results can be obtained with a single film changer and an excellent fluoroscope. In obese patients, the guidewire may be lost in the quantum noise of a poor image intensifier. Very high-resolution television systems (1200 lines) and DSA roadmapping provide an advantage in difficult cases. Intravenous DSA is only indicated when it is not possible or practical to perform an arterial study because the results are poor and significant renal artery lesions can be overlooked. Unless otherwise stated, DSA refers to arterial DSA.

A rate-controlled mechanical injector is necessary for aortic injections and venography. Hand injections are sufficient for selective renal arterial studies.

In cases where renal artery blood flow is high, for example, arteriovenous malformation, a mechanical injector may be needed for selective studies. The radiation dose to the operator is higher with hand injections and all reasonable precautions should be taken including the use of lead glasses and a thyroid shield.

Digital subtraction angiography has a much higher contrast resolution achieved at a measurable loss of spatial resolution than conventional film techniques. However, when fine detail is needed, magnification conventional film series are better (Fig. 9.2). Renal lesions may be missed on aortography and if suspected, selective studies must always be done. A circular field of view (most DSA and film camera examinations) carries the potential risk of missing peripheral renal lesions.

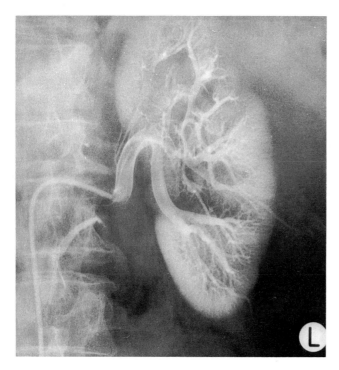

Fig. 9.2 Normal selective renal arteriogram.
Note that the interlobular vessels are clearly seen arising from the arcuate arteries. There is a cortical infarct at the upper pole in which the inter lobular vessels are missing. × 1.64.

RENAL ARTERIAL ANATOMY

The renal arteries arise from the aorta at the level of the first lumbar vertebra. Most often, they are single and pass laterally and horizontally to the renal hilum. The right renal artery is longer and tends to have a more oblique and inferior course than the left. In males, the renal artery has a diameter between 6 and 9 mm and in females between 5 and 8 mm . Each vessel divides into a larger anterior and smaller posterior branch close to the kidney. In 80% of cases, the anterior branch supplies the lower pole and the ventral intermediate portion of the parenchyma. The posterior renal artery supplies the apical and posterior intermediate portion of the parenchyma (Fig. 9.3).

Multiple renal arteries can be expected in 20–30% of patients. The most common arrangement is a small lower pole branch arising from the aorta below the main renal artery or from the ipsilateral iliac artery. Small accessory vessels can be easily overlooked on aortograms. Aberrant branches may occasionally arise from the inferior mesenteric or phrenic arteries. Where malignancy extends into Gerota's

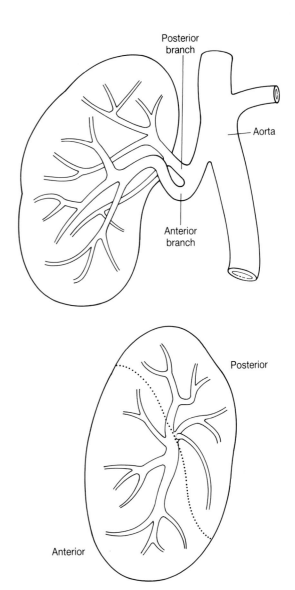

Fig. 9.3 Schematic diagram of the segmental anatomy of the renal circulation.
Variations in the supply to the lower pole are common.

fascia or where there is occlusion of the main renal artery, the kidney may be supplied by adjacent intercostal, lumbar or ureteric vessels. All renal arteries are end arteries and significant trauma to them will render that segment of the kidney ischaemic.

During contrast injection, the renal cortex will be densely and briefly opacified by contrast medium in the capillaries. The subsequent density of the parenchyma is produced by contrast medium first within the tubular epithelium and then within the tubular lumen and collecting tubules of the renal papillae. This will be prolonged by hypotension.

The renal veins are usually poorly seen unless there is poor renal function or a large dose of contrast medium has been used. Unlike the arteries, the renal

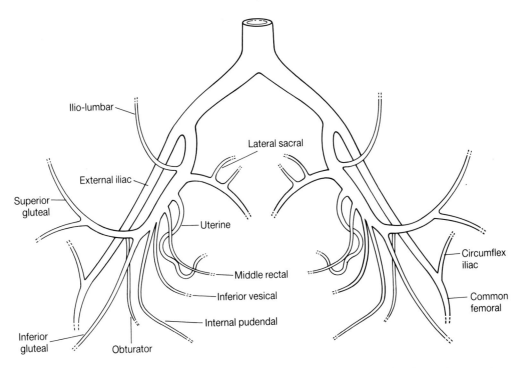

Fig. 9.4 Schematic diagram of the branches of the internal iliac artery (in a hermaphrodite since they have a large uterine artery and a large internal pudendal artery). Variations are common in the internal iliac branches and diagrams such as these are only an approximate guide.

veins intercommunicate freely. Renal venography depends upon this fortunate anatomical arrangement.

The internal iliac artery is a short vessel (4 cm long) which divides into anterior and posterior divisions at the level of the lumbosacral junction. The posterior division divides into the superior gluteal, iliolumbar and two lateral sacral arteries and is the larger of the divisions (Fig. 9.4). The anterior division divides into the superior vesical, obturator, inferior vesical (vaginal), uterine, middle rectal, internal pudendal and inferior gluteal arteries. The major blood supply to the sciatic nerve arises from the inferior gluteal artery below the border of piriformis and embolization of the inferior gluteal should be avoided if the emboli used will occlude distal branches. The uterine artery may arise as a common trunk with the vaginal and middle rectal arteries. It is normally tortuous and runs across the lateral border of the uterus giving branches to the azygos arteries of the vagina, fallopian tube and ovary. The distal tubal branches freely anastomose with the terminal branches of the ovarian artery. The internal pudendal artery exits the pelvis through the greater sciatic foramen, crosses the ischial spine and enters the perineum to divide into the deep and dorsal arteries of the penis. The dorsal artery supplies the glans penis and the deep artery runs forward in the corpora cavernosa. The artery of the urethral bulb is a short vessel of large calibre and supplies the urethral bulb and bulbo-urethral gland.

EXAMINATION TECHNIQUE

Abdominal aortic flush angiography

Catheter: Pigtail (Cook; HN5.0–38–70–P–10S–PIG)
Contrast: Iopromide (Schering AG) or equivalent.
– 300 mgI/ml for DSA: 20–25 ml at 25 ml/sec.
– 370 mgI/m for conventional film: 40–50ml at 25 ml/sec.
Film sequence: 2 per sec for 3 sec
1 per sec for 4 sec

Although the film sequence is the same for either DSA or conventional films, the tendency with DSA is to make many more exposures than is strictly necessary.

CLINICAL INDICATIONS

1 Suspected renal artery stenosis
2 Investigation of renal parenchyma disease including tumours
3 Gross unexplained haematuria
4 Severe renal trauma
5 Prior to interventional procedures, embolization or angioplasty

Aortic flush injections are useful for demonstration of the renal orifice and to provide a roadmap of the renal circulation. The catheter tip should be placed at the level of the superior mesenteric artery. Overlap of the superior mesenteric and renal artery origin is common, but can be avoided by performing the examination with the patient in a slightly oblique position. For surveys in patients with hypertension, both obliques and a single frontal view are obtained.

Selective renal angiography

Catheter: – Cobra 2 (Cook; HNB5.0–35–80–P–NS–C2)
Guidewire: – Cook 0.035 Newton (TSCFNB–35–145–3)or 035 Terumo Angled Glide wire
Contrast: Iopromide (Schering AG) or equivalent 300 mgI/ml for DSA: 10 ml at 8 ml/sec
370 mgI/ml for conventional films: 10 ml/sec
For tumours: 15–25 ml at 10 ml/sec
Film sequence: 2 per sec for 3 sec
1 per sec for 4 sec

The catheter tip must be positioned so that contrast medium will be injected down the vessel rather than against the vessel wall. The contrast volumes specified are only a guide. More diagnoses are missed by inadequate contrast injections than kidneys are damaged by a little more contrast medium.

The right renal artery has a more inferior course from the aorta and may be difficult to catheterize. This can be overcome by inserting a Terumo wire well into the kidney and then advancing the catheter. If this is unsuccessful, then a loop can be made with the cobra catheter (Fig. 9.5), but care must be taken not to allow the catheter tip to penetrate too far down the renal artery or superselective studies will be obtained because the catheter tip is beyond the first branches of the renal artery, usually the posterior branch. A loop is useful to prevent catheter recoil during injection. Alternatively, a catheter with a precurved tip (e.g. a Simmons 2 or 3) may be used.

Adrenaline-enhanced renal angiography is no longer routinely performed as angiography is less critical in the diagnosis of renal masses. If used, a dose of 5–8 μg is injected intra-arterially about 15 sec before the injection of contrast medium for the film run. A much slower rate of injection is needed to avoid damaging the renal artery. With selective injections, it is doubtful if any additional information is obtained with the use of adrenalin (Fig. 9.6). Adrenaline injection is mandatory for renal venography (see Chapter 11).

Selective Adrenal Angiography

Catheter: Cobra 2 (Cook; HNB5.0–35–80–P–NS–C2)
Guidewire: Cook 0.035 (Newton TSCFNB–35–145–3) or Terumo Angled Glide wire
Contrast: Iopromide (Schering AG) or equivalent 300 mg I/ml for DSA: 2–4 ml by hand
370 mgI/ml for conventional films: 4–6 ml by hand
Film sequence: 2 per sec for 3 sec
1 per sec for 4 sec

The adrenal glands are supplied by three small arteries. The upper one usually arises from the inferior phrenic artery and the lower one from the ipsilateral renal artery. The middle one arises directly from the aorta. Since arteriography is performed when the adrenal glands are enlarged by tumour or hyperplasia, arteriography is not as hard as it may seem. If the arteries are very small, a Hilal spinal curve catheter with a tapered tip may be worth trying. If phaeochromocytoma is suspected, adequate premedication is essential to avoid a hypertensive crisis. They may be multiple and arise anywhere along the sympathetic chain. Pelvic tumours are usually adequately demonstrated on a pelvic arteriogram with the catheter tip just above the aortic bifurcation.

Selective gonadal arteriography

Catheter: Rosch Inferior Mesenteric (Cook; BPS6.5–38–80–P–NS–RIM)
Guidewire: Cook 035 TSCFNB–35–145–3 Newton 0.035 Newton or Terumo Angled Glide wire
Contrast: Iopromide (Schering AG) or equivalent 300 mgI/ml for DSA: 2–4 ml by hand
370 mgI/ml for conventional film: at 2 ml/sec
Film sequence 1 per sec for 10 sec

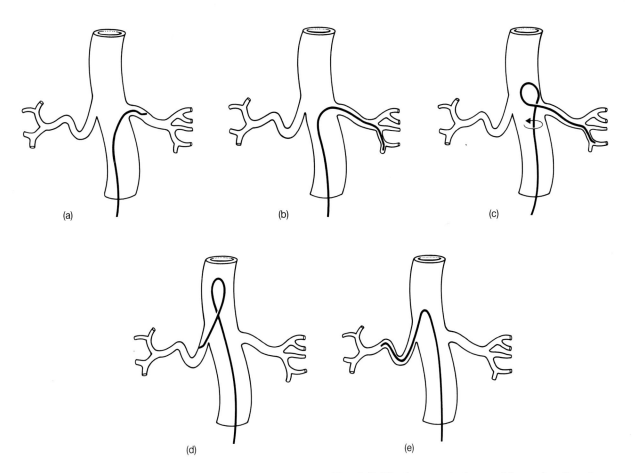

(a)   (b)   (c)

(d)   (e)

Fig. 9.5 The loop technique with a cobra 2 catheter.
In this example, the loop is formed in the left renal artery (a,b,c) and
the loop is used to facilitate deep catheterization of a downward
seeking right renal artery (d,e).

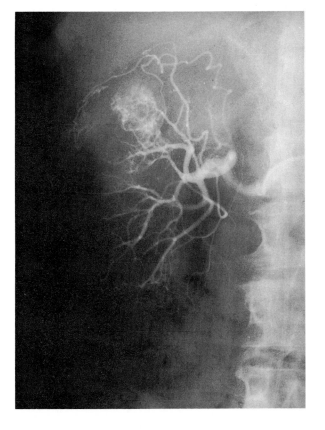

Fig. 9.6 Selective renal arteriography after adrenaline
injection to improve enhancement of tumour vessels.
A reduced injection rate is mandatory to avoid damage to the renal
artery.

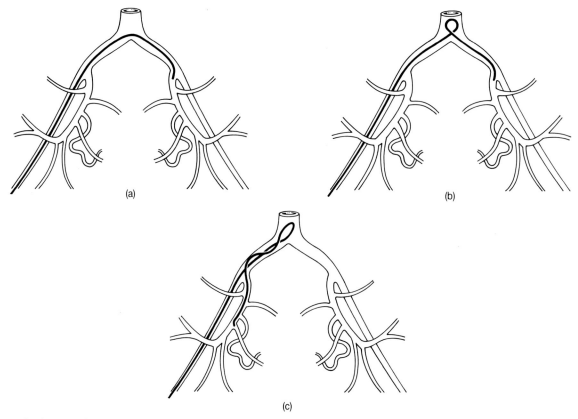

(a)

(b)

(c)

Fig. 9.7 The loop technique for pelvic arteriography.
The loop is formed in the contralateral internal iliac artery (b) and used to facilitate catheterization of the ipsilateral artery (c). The loop may also be formed in the external iliac artery to facilitate catheterization of the contralateral internal iliac artery when this is difficult. Exactly the same technique may be used in the iliac veins.

The gonadal arteries arise from the aorta antero-laterally below the level of the renal arteries and are very difficult to locate. The Rosch Inferior Mesenteric (RIM) catheter has a very small curve at its tip and will locate in a small downward angled branch reliably. This catheter is also appropriate for the inferior mesenteric, hence it's name. There are almost no indications for this examination as US is so good in this region. In females, the ovarian circulation can usually be defined by selective uterine angiography as there is a branch to the ovary along the top of the broad ligament, the tubo-ovarian artery.

Selective internal iliac arteriography

Catheter: Cobra 2 (Cook; HNB5.0–35–80–P–NS–C2)
Guidewire: Cook 0.035 TCSFNB–35–145–3 Newton or Terumo Angled Glide wire
Contrast: Iopromide (Schering AG) 300 mg I/ml for DSA: 8–10 ml by hand

370 mgI/ml for conventional films: 15 ml at 8 ml/sec
Film sequence: 2 per sec for 3 sec
1 per sec for 6 sec

In most patients, it is easy to catheterize the contralateral internal iliac artery from the femoral artery using a guidewire and cobra catheter. To catheterize the ipsilateral side, the cobra is made into a loop from the internal iliac on the contralateral side and brought across the bifurcation (Fig. 9.7). Care must be taken in patients with atheroma at the bifurcation as some atheroma may be displaced and emboli will occur distally.

In females, indications for iliac angiography are usually bleeding from the uterus because of arteriovenous malformations or tumour. A single anteroposterior projection is sufficient for investigation. If bleeding is due to tumour, films should include the symphysis as often the obturator branches supply the mass.

In males, the primary indication is impotence. Firstly, the status of the distal aorta and common iliac vessels is assessed by flush aortography. Then, internal pudendal angiography is performed following which 60 mg papaverine is injected directly into the corpora cavernosa or through the catheter directly into the internal pudendal artery. If spasm of the artery occurs, vasodilators (nitroglycerine, tolazoline) are injected intra-arterially or the patient is given an epidural anaesthetic. If the major penile arteries are not seen following internal iliac or more selective studies, then the external pudendal which arises from the common femoral arteries should be injected.

SUGGESTED FURTHER READING

BAHREN W, GALL H, SSHERB W (1988) Arterial anatomy and arteriographic diagnosis of arteriogenic impotence. *Cardiovascular Interventional Radiology* 11: 195.

BOIJSEN E (1959) Angiographic studies of the anatomy of single and multiple renal arteries. *Acta Radiologica(Suppl)* 183: 1.

CRAGG AH, NAKAGAWA N, SMITH TP, BERBAUM KS (1991) Haematoma formation after diagnostic angiography:effect of catheter size. *Journal of Vascular and Interventional Radiology* 2: 231.

HARRIS KG, SMITH TP, CRAGG AH, LEMKE JH (1991) Nephrotoxicity from contrast material in renal insufficiency. *Radiology* 179: 849.

CHAPTER 10

Therapeutic urogenital angiography

Ken R. Thomson and Neale A. Walters

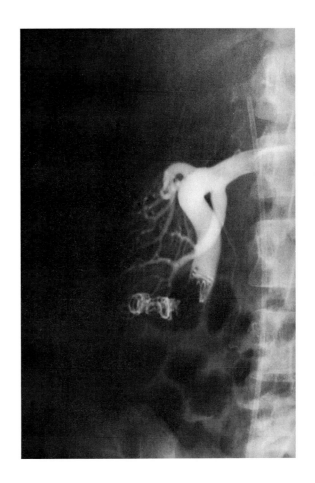

PATIENT PREPARATION

The general comments of Chapter 9 apply for therapeutic angiography. However, some therapeutic procedures are painful and attention must be paid to pain relief both during and after the procedure. Usually, neuroleptanalgesia is sufficient, but in cases where large tumours are embolized, epidural anaesthesia during and for 2–3 days after the procedure gives excellent control over pain. Otherwise, for postprocedural pain, a titrated opiate infusion is ideal, the most effective use of which is when the patients control the dose themselves.

All patients should have an intravenous line inserted and these procedures demand the support and backup of surgical colleagues.

EQUIPMENT OPTIONS

These are described in Chapter 9. These procedures are easier, safer and quicker if digital subtraction angiography (DSA) is used. The ability to display a 'roadmap' quickly in a compound oblique without having to move the patient is desirable.

THERAPEUTIC OPTIONS

Infusion therapy

This involves selective catheterization of the target organ and injection of a therapeutic substance over a period of minutes, hours or days depending on the substance. We have experience of infusion of lymphocyte cultures, monoclonal antibodies and cytotoxic drugs, principally *cis*-platinum for tumour palliation. Such methods have a poor response rate and have been used as a last resort.

For short-term infusions (up to 24 hours) a femoral approach is satisfactory. For long-term infusions, an upper brachial approach is preferable to allow the patient mobility. A 5 Fr catheter with a coaxial 3 Fr catheter is used so that if the catheter becomes occluded with thrombus it can easily be replaced with another. A heparin lock of 5000 IU is injected in the small space left in the outer catheter via a Tuohy Borst adapter. The 3 Fr catheter effectively obturates the tip of the 5 French catheter. An infusion rate of 60 ml/hour will keep the smaller catheter clear and its diameter is small enough not to cause vessel occlusion or thrombosis.

ANGIOPLASTY

Angioplasty is performed in the renal, internal iliac and pudendal arteries. The indications are renovascular hypotension, preservation of renal function and impotence.

Even when there is clear evidence of excessive renin production as the cause of the hypertension, patients are given their normal medication on the day of the procedure. The halflife of renin is about 6 hours and in over 100 renal angioplasties, we have not seen a precipitous fall in blood pressure unless it was caused by fluid depletion.

Vascular surgical consultation is mandatory because of the possible risk of rupture or prolonged and untreatable spasm of the renal artery. If this occurs, an infusion of low molecular weight dextran is started and heparin 5000 IU, is given intravenously. In most cases the kidney will survive for an hour or so until bypass surgery because of collateral arterial supply.

Spasm of a branch renal artery is more common when deep guidewire insertion has occurred, but it responds well to nitroglycerin injections into the renal artery. Embolization with microparticles of cholesterol has been seen on renal biopsy after otherwise uneventful angioplasty. It is usually subclinical, but worsening of pre-existing renal failure is reported. Although there is good evidence of the value of renal angioplasty, iliac or pudendal angioplasty is still to be proved as a treatment for impotence.

RENAL ARTERY ANGIOPLASTY

Indications

The ideal lesion for renal angioplasty is a short segment stenosis in a horizontal vessel with no proximal branches (Fig. 10.1). Since this situation is

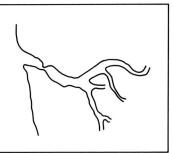

(a) Single simple stenosis

A catheter can be safely sited proximal to the stenosis and a catheter exchange method used. A stent would not be used unless the balloon result was unsatisfactory

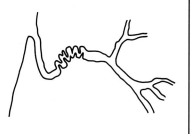

(b) Complex nonorificial stenosis

This is typical of fibromuscular disease. A catheter exchange method may be tried but a coaxial method will have a higher chance of primary success. Stenting would not usually be necessary in fibromuscular disease

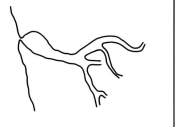

(c) Orificial stenosis

The angiographic catheter will not engage the orifice and the wireguide will be likely to dissect the aortic plaque around the orifice. A coaxial catheter technique and elective stent after angioplasty is recommended

Fig. 10.1 The type of renal artery stenosis determines the angioplasty method most appropriate.

Type (a) lesions are suited to a simple technique whereas type (b) and (c) lesions require more skill.

uncommon, renal angioplasty can be difficult and the results are not as good as femoral or iliac angioplasty.

Fibromuscular hyperplasia generally involves the media and is most common in a ptosed right renal artery. The lesion is a series of baffles or webs, some of which are quite thick and resist the passage of even a steerable guidewire. The lesion dilates easily, however, and the results are usually excellent.

Stenosis due to atheroma involving the origin of the renal artery is complicated by occlusion of the artery during catheter manipulation when atheromatous material from the aorta is pushed into the renal artery. A coaxial system permits a more con-

trolled probing of the origin and contrast injections during guidewire manipulation. These lesions are likely to recur following angioplasty because of the elasticity of the aorta and the inability of a balloon to overcome the elastic recoil without rupture. Recurrent stenoses can be avoided by placing a stent in the renal artery following angioplasty.

Atheromatous stenoses involving the renal artery distal to it's origin, but proximal to the first branch, respond quite well to angioplasty with a similar recurrence rate to femoral angioplasty (25–30%).

Arterial stenosis in the renal transplant is usually at the site of the surgical anastomosis and dilates well unless an end-to-side anastomosis with the external iliac artery has been fashioned.

Techniques

CATHETER EXCHANGE TECHNIQUE

The renal artery is first assessed with flush aortography (Chapter 9). The renal artery is then catheterized with a diagnostic catheter (Cook; HNB5.0–35–80–P–NS–C2) and the stenosis crossed with a tapered straight guidewire with a floppy tip (Cook; TSCFNB–35–145–3 Newton) or an angled tip glide wire (Terumo). The catheter is then advanced over the guidewire past the stenosis. The pressure in the renal artery is compared to that of the aorta. If the stenosis is very tight, the renal artery may be occluded by the catheter with no pulsatile waveform beyond the stenosis. A movable core guidewire (Cook TSCM) with a 1 cm flexible tip is then exchanged for the straight guidewire which usually straightens the renal artery. The tip of this guidewire is quite stiff and can dissect the artery if pushed too hard. Once across the stenosis, the diagnostic catheter is removed and replaced with a balloon (Cook; AXM5–35–80–6–4.0, 6 mm diameter, 4 cm long) of suitable size. The balloon size is determined by the size of the renal artery. Its actual size can be measured with the DSA computer, but if conventional film is being used, the balloon should be matched to the direct measured size of the artery from the film. This gives about a 10% overestimation. Most commonly, a 6 mm diameter balloon is used. Long balloons of 4 cm are ideal as this prevents the balloon moving out of the stenosis as it is inflated. The balloon should not be positioned across arterial bifurcations especially if atheroma is present. Side branches can be occluded by plaque as the balloon is dilated. It does not matter if part of the balloon is in the aorta. Modern angioplasty balloons are not elastic and will not dilate beyond their design diameter.

Once in position, gently inflate the balloon watching the pressure changes within the artery and the fluoroscopic image and inflate until the constriction on the balloon disappears or the patient feels pain. It is normal for the patient to feel slight discomfort during angioplasty, which should disappear immediately with deflation of the balloon. A long inflation time is not required. Flush the catheter between inflations to avoid thrombus in the catheter gently as vigorously flushing may lift a dissection at the angioplasty site. Measure the arterial pressure in the renal artery as the catheter is withdrawn. The residual gradient should be less than 10–15 mm Hg.

Films after angioplasty are obtained either with the balloon catheter close to the orifice or by aortography. If the result is unsatisfactory then the procedure can be repeated with a bigger angioplasty catheter. Beware of using too large a balloon as the danger of rupture of the renal artery can occur, even when a lower pressure is used. The force exerted on the arterial wall is a function of the balloon surface area as well as the inflation pressure.

If the procedure is complicated by renal artery rupture, then the patient will complain of flank or back pain and contrast medium will extravasate. The conventional wisdom is to inflate the balloon in the renal artery to stop the leak and call for your vascular surgeon. This assumes firstly that surgical backup is available and secondly that there is some renal artery stump in which to inflate the balloon.

The exchange method is simple, cheap and quick. This is the procedure beginners should master first before tackling coaxial procedures and transplant angioplasty. Unless there is scar tissue or Dacron in the puncture site a sheath is not required.

Normally heparin is not given when a short procedural time is expected, but 2500 IU gives a measure of safety and the puncture site compression time is not significantly prolonged by this low dose.

COAXIAL ANGIOPLASTY

This technique employs an 8 Fr guide catheter (Schneider), a coaxial 5 Fr angioplasty catheter (Schneider Winning set) and a steerable 0.014 inch guidewire. If a stent insertion is planned, ensure that it will fit through the guide catheter first (a 9 Fr guide catheter is required for a Palmaz stent). The guide catheter has a soft and rather blunt tip and must be inserted through a sheath. Intravenous or intra-arterial heparin 5000 IU, is given once the sheath is inserted and 10 ml nitroglycerin in a dose of 100 µg/ml is prepared in case of spasm in the renal artery. The heparin is given because the guidewire will be left through the angioplasty catheter for most of the procedure and although the catheter can be flushed through a Tuohy Borst adapter, there is a higher risk of thrombus than with an empty catheter.

The guide catheter is positioned adjacent to the renal artery orifice and the stenosis identified clearly by injections of contrast medium. The stenosis is crossed with the steerable guidewire, the angioplasty catheter is advanced across the stenosis and inflated. The process can be monitored at any time by an injection of contrast medium through the guide catheter which is the advantage of this technique. Simultaneous arterial pressure measurements may also be obtained from the guide catheter in the aorta and by the angioplasty catheter in the renal artery.

If the stenosis is very tight and the angioplasty catheter will not cross the stenosis, attempts to advance it will push the guide catheter away from the orifice and the guidewire will buckle out of the renal artery. The reason for this is that the flexible tip of the guidewire is too long. This can be overcome if a shorter floppy tip guidewire (target therapeutics) is used. The mandril of the Stubby wire will now support the angioplasty catheter across the stenosis. The disadvantage of the Stubby wire is that it is more likely to damage the renal artery distally as it is stiffer.

If the renal artery lesion is bilateral, then a coaxial technique is preferred because it makes changes of catheter easier. The disadvantage of the coaxial technique is firstly that a 9 Fr sheath is needed and secondly that the largest diameter balloon that can be used is 6 mm , which is usually big enough for renal arteries.

Should spasm occur during angioplasty, nitroglycerin is given directly into the renal artery in 100–200 µg aliquots through the guide catheter.

RENAL TRANSPLANT ARTERY ANGIOPLASTY

In transplanted kidneys, there is no collateral supply and because it is denervated, no sensation of pressure as the balloon is inflated. These features increase the risk of transplant angioplasty, but in practise the stenoses are usually easier to dilate than in the native vessels. The exchange technique is all that is required.

INTERNAL ILIAC AND PUDENDAL ARTERY ANGIOPLASTY

These vessels are most easily dilated from the contralateral side using an exchange technique. If angioplasty is being performed for impotence, it is only likely to succeed if both sides are diseased. Only one functioning pudendal artery is required for erection to occur.

Spasm is a common complication of small vessel angioplasty. Nitroglycerin is administered prior to angioplasty as a sublingual tablet or as a paste placed on the patient's skin. It is far easier to prevent arterial spasm than to reduce spasm once it has been developed.

RENAL ARTERY STENT INSERTION

Renal artery stents are used to maintain patency when there is:

1 Elastic recoil
2 Dissection that threatens patency
3 A gradient of more than 10–15 mm Hg after angioplasty

There are two types of stent: balloon expandable (Palmaz) or self-expanding (Wallstent, Strecker). These involve an additional level of complexity, but offer the hope of prolonged patency and less restenosis particularly for orificial lesions.

Insertion techniques differ, but with all types of stent it is essential to ensure that it is accurately positioned (Fig. 10.2).

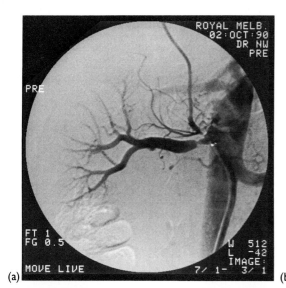

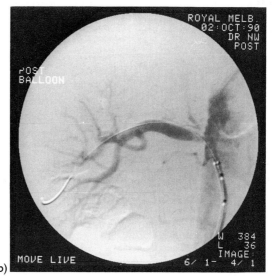

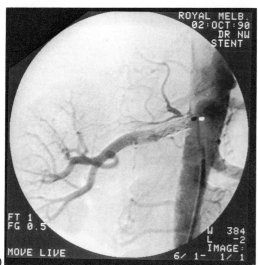

Fig. 10.2 Renal angioplasty and stent insertion.
(a) An irregular lesion close to the orifice of the renal artery prior to angioplasty. The guide catheter has a opaque ring at its tip which allows accurate measurement of the renal artery diameter. (b) After angioplasty, there is a residual stenosis. The guidewire has been left across the stenosis, an advantage of the coaxial technique. (c) After Palmaz stent insertion at the angioplasty site. The stenosis is completely relieved and no residual arterial pressure gradient was detected.

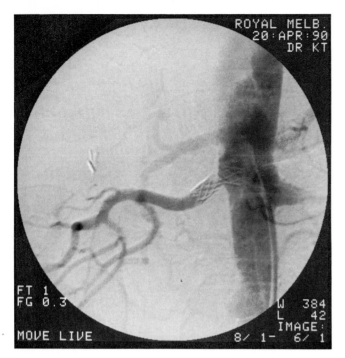

Fig. 10.3 Poor placement of an articulated Palmaz renal artery stent.
The articulation is situated at the renal artery orifice and as a result, the stenosis is poorly relieved and too much of the stent projects into the aorta. Once deployed, it is not possible to remove without open surgery.

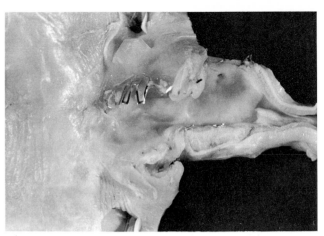

Fig. 10.4 Neointimal lining of a Palmaz renal artery stent.
This patient died from unrelated causes 6 months after stent insertion. The internal surface of the stent has been almost completely covered except where the stent projects into the aorta. Neointimal overgrowth is a cause of restenosis and is more commonly seen in smaller vessels.

The Palmaz stent should be positioned with the end of the stent projecting about 1.5 mm into the aorta. The stent is deployed by inflation of the balloon. Once deployed, it cannot be moved. If the stent is a little loose on the balloon catheter it may slide back as the stent is advanced into the renal artery. It can be pushed back into position with a guide catheter tip as long as the balloon has not been inflated. The Palmaz stent is rigid and provides the best looking poststent appearances (Fig. 10.3).

The Strecker stent and the Wallstent are self-expanding.

A follow-up arteriogram at 6 months is performed to confirm patency. Intravenous DSA and Doppler ultrasound do not provide sufficient detail to exclude intimal proliferation within the stent. Intrastent stenosis can be treated by balloon angioplasty (Fig. 10.4).

If a stent migrates distally, leave the angioplasty guidewire through the stent and remove the angioplasty catheter with which it was inserted. Insert a stone basket retrieval catheter into the guide catheter alongside the guidewire and grasp the stent in the basket. The original guidewire will keep the stent from floating off with the blood flow. Once the stent has been ensnared and the basket closed around it, it will collapse sufficiently to be safely withdrawn to the puncture site.

EMBOLIC MATERIALS

Gelfoam

Gelfoam is presented in sheets 2 cm wide and 4 cm long. It is delivered either as a slurry or as a torpedo.

To make a slurry, gently tease the Gelfoam apart with a scalpel until about one-third to one-half of the sheet is used. Cut off the distal half of the tip of a plastic 2ml syringe, withdraw the plunger and place the dry Gelfoam chips in the syringe with a pair of forceps. Mix the Gelfoam with 1.5 ml contrast medium and shake the syringe vigorously.

Torpedoes are made from a triangular slice made across the long axis of the Gelfoam pad and rolled tightly between the thumb and index finger. Half fill a 2 ml syringe with contrast and aspirate some air. Insert the torpedo thin end first with a twisting motion and hold it in position with your finger as the air is expelled slowly. The torpedo can be injected with the 2 ml syringe, but if catheter recoil is a problem load the torpedo with a gentle injection of the 2ml syringe and expel it from the catheter with a 1 ml syringe.

Coils

Coils are lengths of guidewire springs in various configurations with woollen or Dacron (e.g. Cook MWCE–38–5–8) threads attached to cause thrombosis. Special sizes and shapes can be ordered from the manufacturer to suit a particular application. The coils work best when they are arranged radially around the arterial wall and mechanically occluding much of the flow. In practise this hardly ever happens. If the diameter of the coil is too large for the vessel, the coil will wind along the vessel and not produce a good effect. It is also more likely to extrude along the vessel. If the coil is too small, it will float distally with blood flow. As embolization is established, blood flow may reverse or eddy such that a small coil floats back into the access vessel.

Coils are relatively easy to grasp with a wire snare and retrieve via a sheath. In cases of arteriovenous malformations with very high flow the coils may be inserted through an occlusion balloon catheter which will reduce or stop the blood flow to the organ (Fig. 10.5). If the delivery catheter flicks out of the artery as soon as the coil starts to extrude from it, it is best to stop the delivery and retrieve the coil while you still have part of it inside the delivery catheter.

A mixture of Gelfoam and coils is very effective in renal tumours for preoperative reduction of blood supply.

Particles

Particulate emboli of various sizes are available in a wide range of materials including plastics, iron microspheres and collagen. These are more suited for arteriovenous malformations and tumours where an occlusion balloon catheter cannot be used. They are mixed with contrast medium in a small dish to make them visible as negative filling defects and injected using a 2ml syringe. Ivalon (polyvinyl alcohol foam) particles are visible by computed tomography (CT) because they are impregnated with barium. Under fluoroscopy most particles are not opaque and check injections of contrast medium should be made to see that reflux of contrast medium (and particles) is not occurring. A Gelfoam torpedo injected after the particles will help clear the catheter of stray particles.

Liquids

For tumour palliation absolute alcohol, Ethibloc and Histoacryl (N-butylcyanoacrylate) are more effec-

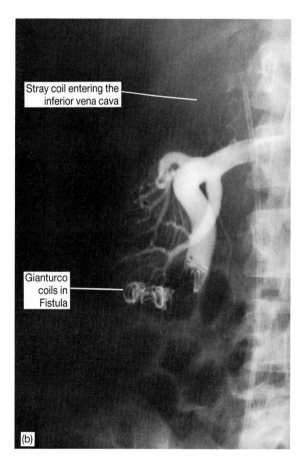

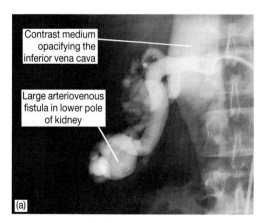

Fig. 10.5 Coil occlusion of a large renal arteriovenous fistula due to a renal biopsy in a patient with high output cardiac failure.
(a) Preliminary angiography shows a large varix at the lower pole (bottom arrow) with rapid a dense opacification of the inferior vena cava (top arrow). (b) Several large Gianturco coils (bottom arrow) have been inserted into the fistula using an occlusion balloon to reduce the flow through the fistula. In spite of this, a single coil extruded into the inferior vena cava (top arrow) which was removed with a wire snare.

tive since these compounds also occlude the collateral supply to the tumour.

Balloon occlusion catheters are mandatory for the use of absolute alcohol and recommended with Ethibloc. Once the access artery has been occluded by the balloon, contrast medium is injected to fill completely the circulation to be embolized. This is the maximum volume of the liquid which should be injected. The agent is injected with the balloon inflated and left to 'soak' for 2–3 min before the balloon is deflated. A further injection of contrast medium is made to check results. Ethibloc is a radio-opaque alcoholic suspension of corn protein with a consistency of clear honey (Fig. 10.6). It is injected with a 1 ml syringe as it is quite viscous. The occlusion balloon is left inflated for 5 min. Ethibloc can also be injected through a Cook Explorer 2.6 Fr coaxial catheter which has been placed highly selectively. In this situation Ethibloc acts in a similar fashion to tissue adhesives except that the catheter will not be glued in place.

Histoacryl (*N*-butyl cyanoacrylate) is a tissue adhesive which is currently under a suspicion of oncogenicity even though no evidence of this has been found in the many patients who have been embolized with this material. The Histoacryl polymerizes exothermically in contact with free ionic radicals in the mixture. A 3 Fr coaxial catheter is used for delivery and the catheters should be flushed with 5% dextrose prior to injection. To make the Histoacryl radio-opaque and to retard it's polymerization, it is mixed with Ultrafluid Lipiodol in a Histoacryl to Lipiodol ratio of 1:2. This gives a polymerization time of about 5 sec. The volume of the coaxial catheter and stopcock is determined and using a three-way stopcock, the catheter is first flushed with 5% dextrose, filled with Histoacryl to less than the volume of the catheter so that the Histoacryl is entirely within the catheter. Five per cent dextrose is then injected to push the Histoacryl out of the catheter as it is withdrawn. The catheter is removed to avoid gluing the catheter to the artery wall or to avoid pulling the embolus out with the catheter.

The choice of embolic material is sometimes determined by the patient's anatomy and inability to place a suitable catheter safely for the embolic material which was originally planned to be used.

INDICATIONS FOR UROGENITAL ARTERIAL EMBOLIZATION

1 Control of bleeding
2 Treatment of arteriovenous malformations and fistulae
3 Ablation of function
4 Palliation of malignant tumours

RENAL ARTERY EMBOLIZATION

If the embolization is for preoperative reduction in blood supply to a renal tumour, then the procedure should be performed the day before surgery to minimize the patient's pain. Catheterize the renal artery and check that the catheter position is stable by inserting a straight wire guide through the catheter and by making a forceful injection of contrast medium. When the position is stable, fill the renal artery with Gelfoam and put a coil at the origin of the first branch. Leave room for a surgical clamp around the proximal renal artery. The main value of embolization in the preoperative situation is that it will cause deflation of the large draining veins from the tumour. These are more of a problem for the surgeon than the artery. Resist the temptation to place a large coil in the main access artery if there is a probability that you will need to repeat the embolization later. Collaterals may open up which cannot be catheterized.

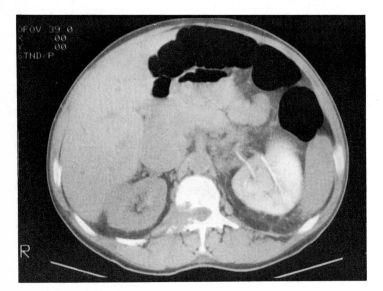

Fig. 10.6 Renal artery embolization with Ethibloc to control haematuria in advanced renal malignancy.
A computed tomographic scan taken after the procedure shows almost complete filling of the left renal circulation with Ethibloc. There is a metastasis in a vertebral body.

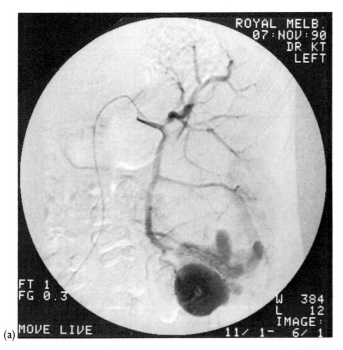

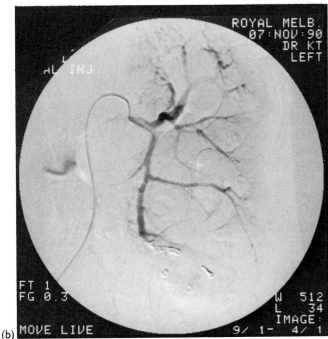

For a small arteriovenous malformation or a fistula, try and place the catheter tip in the feeding vessels to minimize damage to the kidney. A 3 Fr coaxial catheter (Cook Explorer, Target Tracker–18) makes superselective catheterization much easier. Microcoils which fit through the 3 Fr catheter can be placed very accurately and particles are not usually necessary. Embolization should be as selective as possible to preserve the normal renal parenchyma (Fig. 10.7). Histoacryl may be indicated in an arteriovenous malformation to occlude the nidus, but it should be given with extreme care. If the catheter tip does become glued in place, advance the outer catheter as far as possible and tug on the inner catheter sharply. Usually either the catheter will free itself or it will break off close to the tip where the catheter is softest. The small piece of tubing left in the distal renal artery may thrombose, but it will probably be covered with intima in a few weeks. It is not worth worrying about unless the viability of the entire kidney is threatened.

If the procedure is for traumatic haemorrhage, then complete capillary occlusion is unwarranted and a few plugs of Gelfoam are all that are required.

For tumour palliation, Ethibloc gives more predictable results. As the tumours are likely to be large, angiography of the adjacent intercostal and lumbar vessels which may supply the lesion is performed and if necessary, embolized with small Ivalon particles or Ethibloc using a coaxial catheter (Fig. 10.8).

Fig. 10.7 Superselective renal artery embolization.
(a) A patient with bilateral angiomyolipoma had a kidney removed because of suspected tumour presented with recurrent severe haematuria. The initial angiogram shows a large varix at the lower pole with stretching of the arteries in the middle portion of the kidney from the tumour. (b) After embolization with microcoils through a 2.5 Fr coaxial catheter, only the varix has been embolized with preservation of the two small arteries to the functioning lower pole parenchyma.

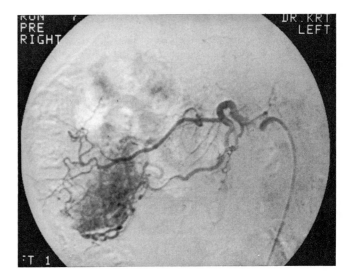

Fig. 10.8 Lumbar artery supply to a renal carcinoma.
Selective injection into the right lumbar artery shows extensive neovascularity at the site of the renal tumour. This was embolized using a 2.6 Fr coaxial catheter and Ethibloc. The anterior spinal artery must not be occluded.

EMBOLIZATION OF THE ADRENAL GLANDS

Indications for adrenal embolization are to palliate tumours or control secretion of hormones, specifically cortisol. Either the three supplying arteries or the single draining vein can be embolized. Vein occlusion is a complication of adrenal venography and can be occluded by over-injecting the adrenal vein with hot contrast medium with the intention of destroying the gland. Arterial occlusion is best achieved with Ivalon particles.

EMBOLIZATION OF THE TESTICULAR VEIN

This technique has become popular as an alternative to surgical ligation of the testicular vein in the treatment of oligospermia and infertility related to a varicocoele and also to symptomatic varicocoeles with normal fertility. The veins are embolized using coils at the pelvic brim and close to the outlet of the vein with the inferrior vena cava (IVC) on the right and with the renal vein on the left. Detachable balloons and Amplatz Spiders (Cook) can be used to prevent migration of the coils from the vein.

The left testicular vein is usually easily accessed from the femoral route with a cobra 2 catheter and floppy tip guidewire (Cook TSCFNB–35–145–3 Newton). Alternatively to coils, hot contrast medium and sclerosants, for example, sodium tetradecyl sulphate (Sotradechol) have been injected with the patient performing the Valsalva manouevre to prevent reflux into the IVC. Complications include pulmonary embolisation of coils and testicular phleboliths. These are fortunately infrequent but care should be taken to prevent any sclerosant material from reaching the pampiniform plexus.

A repeat venogram should be performed about 15–20 min after embolization to check the results and position of coils.

EMBOLIZATION OF THE INTERNAL ILIAC ARTERY

Indications are:

1 Haemorrhage following trauma or due to pelvic malignancy
2 Priapism

Haemorrhage following trauma usually responds to a syringe or two of Gelfoam slurry into the proximal internal iliac artery on the side of bleeding or bilaterally. There is a significant risk of ischaemic damage to the sciatic nerve if the inferior gluteal branch of the internal iliac artery is embolized. The Gelfoam slurry will not occlude the collaterals upon which the blood supply to the sciatic nerve depends when the internal iliac artery is occluded. Collaterals to the inferior gluteal arise from the cruciate anastomosis supplied from the circumflex femoral branch of the profunda femoris artery. If small particles or liquids are used in the pelvis, then the inferior gluteal artery should be protected by an occlusion balloon or even a large proximal Gelfoam plug.

Similarly for bleeding from advanced malignancy, Gelfoam slurry will often be sufficient. If possible the catheter tip should be placed into the uterine or vesical arteries rather than just the anterior division of the internal iliac artery before emboli are injected. Even after radiotherapy this can safely be done bilaterally. The patients are tired, sick and frightened and the simplest, quickest procedure which will stop the bleeding is indicated.

A more selective embolization is indicated for an arteriovenous malformation of the uterus in a young female who wants to have a pregnancy. In such situations, Ivalon particles, 500 microns in diameter, are injected to reduce the vascularity of the uterus. Even with a successful embolization, the risk of exsanguination with a subsequent pregnancy is significant.

Priapism which is resistant to other forms of treatment, such as aspiration of the corpora cavernosa or shunts to the spongiosa, may require embolization of the pudendal artery. This should be done as selectively as possible with a single Gelfoam torpedo. If a 3 Fr catheter is used which will not accept a torpedo, then the catheter can be left to fill with autologous clot and then flushed with a 1 ml syringe. This is the only time we recommend autologous clot as it is too unpredictable and clumsy to use compared to the other materials described above.

PENILE VENOABLATION

This technique is indicated for impotence due to venous leakage. Catheterize the dorsal vein of the penis, select the draining veins one by one and occlude them with small coils. Finally the dorsal vein should be occluded. This should stop the leak and allow normal penile function. In practise, it is difficult to catheterize the dorsal vein without surgical exposure and the number of veins to be occluded is large. An alternative retrograde approach from the iliac veins has been proposed, but the catheter is hard to manipulate across the myriad of valves in the pudendal vein. Our personal experience with either technique is so far disappointing.

POSTEMBOLIZATION CARE

Whenever a significant mass of tissue is embolized, the patient will experience a 'post-infarction' syndrome. This comprises pain, fever and elevation of the white cell count. The pain usually begins within 15–20 min after the embolization and persists for 1–2 days. Postembolization pain is reduced when local anaesthetic is injected just prior to the embolization or when absolute alcohol is used. Absolute alcohol is intensely painful for 2–3 min after injection.

Within 24 hours, gas bubbles will appear in the infarcted tissue. This is less noticeable after the use of liquids and Ethibloc in particular and we believe it is due to release of nitrogen from vessels in the area of infarction. When Ethibloc is used it is infused under pressure until it completely flushes out all the blood and this is probably why gas is less often seen. The only problem with the gas is that it mimics gas-producing infection. In such cases the area of infarction swells much more rapidly and the patient is clearly ill. Serial CT scans are helpful in this regard.

In large tumours, an epidural anaesthetic for 2–3 days postembolization is very effective. Superselective embolization of tumour vessels is sometimes quite painless.

SUGGESTED FURTHER READING

BOOKSTEIN JJ, LURIE AL (1988) Transluminal penile vasoablation for impotence: a progress report. *Cardiovascular and Interventional Radiology* **168**: 137.

GRIMM CE, WHITWORTH JA, THOMSOM KR, HARE WSC, KINCAID-SMITH PKS (1958) Treatment of renal artery stenosis with percutaneous transluminal angioplasty. *Australian Radiology* **29**: 42.

KLINGE MD, WILLEM PTM, MALI MD, PUILJAERT CBAJ, GESYKES GG, BECKING WB, FELDBERG MAM (1989) Percutaneous transluminal renal angioplasty: initial and long term results. *Radiology* **171**: 501.

ZEITLER E, JECHT E, RICHTER EL, SEYFERTH W (1980) Selective sclerotherapy of the internal spermatic vein in patients with varicoceoles. *Cardiovascular Interventional Radiology* **3**: 166.

Urogenital venography

Neale A. Walters and Ken R. Thomson

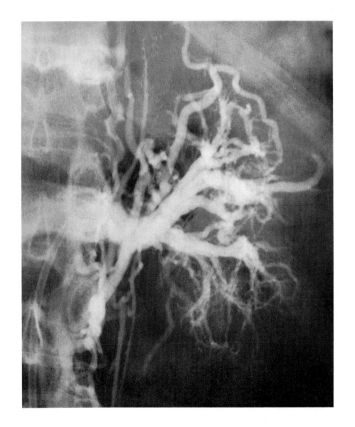

PATIENT PREPARATION

Preparation is the same as for renal angiography (Chapter 9). If venous sampling is to be performed, renin antagonists should be withdrawn for 2 days before the procedure and adrenal sampling should be done in the morning. The volume of blood needed for analysis and the preparation of it must be checked with the biochemistry department. The indications for venography are:

1 Renal vein thrombosis
2 Renal vein sampling for renin (hypertension)
3 Adrenal vein sampling
4 Testicular venography (varicocoele, cryptorchidism)
5 Ovarian venography (pelvic congestion syndrome and venous sampling)

As with renal angiography, high-quality fluoroscopy, preferably digital subtraction angiography (DSA), nonionic contrast medium and a mechanical injector are needed.

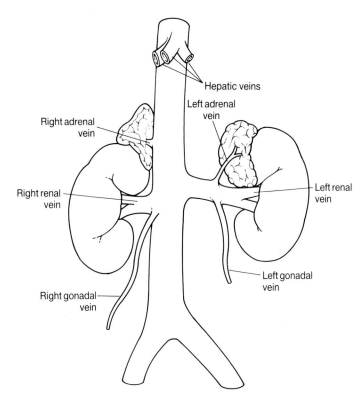

Fig. 11.1 Schematic diagram of the inferior vena cava and its major tributaries.

RENAL VENOUS ANATOMY

Both main renal veins enter the inferior vena cava (IVC) at a level between the first and third lumbar vertebrae. The right renal vein is shorter than the left and passes inferiorly and laterally from the IVC. The right testicular vein enters the IVC just inferior and anterior to the entry of the right renal vein. The right adrenal vein, which may occasionally be multiple, enters the IVC superiorly and slightly posteriorly to the renal vein. The left renal vein receives the left adrenal vein on its superior aspect and the left spermatic vein on its inferior aspect (Fig. 11.1). The renal and adrenal veins do not have valves, but there is a valve at the orifice of the gonadal vein.

The left renal vein usually passes between the aorta and superior mesenteric artery, but may be retroaortic or occasionally duplicated passing anterior and posterior to the aorta. The retroaortic renal vein may arise significantly lower than the right renal vein. When the left renal vein forms a venous ring around the aorta the adrenal vein originates from the upper portion of the ring and the gonadal vein from the lower portion (Fig. 11.2). The renal vein tributaries freely anastomose within the kidneys.

The spermatic veins may have multiple duplicated segments and may anastomose freely with the lumbar veins.

EXAMINATION TECHNIQUE

Initial venepuncture

The IVC is entered via the femoral vein unless contraindicated (lower IVC occlusion, IVC filter, bilateral iliac vein occlusions) when the catheter can be introduced via the brachial or jugular veins. If the brachial vein is large, this is an easy route for diagnostic venography and renin sampling. Puncture of the internal jugular vein is technically more difficult and carries a small risk of air embolism. It should be performed in a head-dependent (Trendelenberg) position.

Puncture of the femoral vein is performed at the level of the inguinal crease. Palpate the femoral artery and after injection of local anaesthetic, insert the puncture needle (Cook; SDN–18–7.0) just medial to the artery. The femoral vein is punctured with

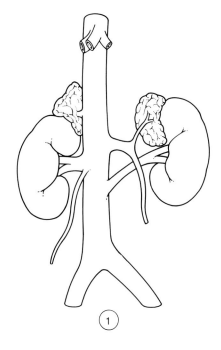

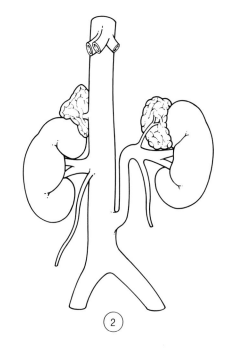

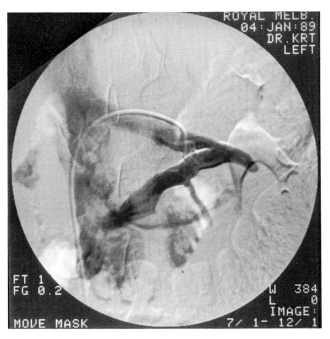

Fig. 11.2 Renal vein anomalies.
(a1) Schematic diagram showing a retroaortic left renal vein due to persistence of the left supracardinal vein. In this diagram the left adrenal and gonadal veins arise normally from the intersubcardinal venous anastomosis. (a2) Low junction point of the left renal vein and inferior vena cava. This is due to persistence of a low intersupracardinal anastomosis. The adrenal and gonadal veins arise from the left renal vein normally. (b) Venogram showing a left renal venous ring with an upper preaortic segment and a lower retroartic segment. The gonadal vein can be seen arising from the lower component of the ring.

the single part needle connected to a plastic 10 ml syringe. With practise puncture of the vein can be felt as a 'pop' and aspiration will result in free egress of venous blood. Asking the patient to bear down or perform a Valsalva manouevre is not necessary when a sharp needle is used. A small 'J' tip guidewire (Cook; TSCF–35–145–1.5) is introduced through the needle and the catheter inserted over the guidewire. The same needle and guidewire techniques are used for jugular or brachial punctures.

If more than one venous catheter is required, then a further puncture may be made in the same femoral vein a little lower than the first puncture. If the puncture is made above the first one, place a guidewire in the first catheter to avoid cutting the catheter with a needle (this is not really a problem with wire-braided catheters).

A variety of catheters can be used, but the most useful is the Cobra 2 (Cook; HBP5.5–38–80–M–NS–C2). Numerous proprietary shapes are available, for example, right and left selective renal vein curves, but if a loop technique is used with the cobra (see Chapter 10), then a single catheter is needed.

It is advisable to fashion a second hole in the side of the catheter near its tip to prevent the tip of the catheter from obstructing on the wall of the vein as suction is applied for sampling (Cook; HPFTS–100 hole punch set). Take care not to make the side hole too far from the tip because veins like the right adrenal vein are short and it may result in blood being incorrectly sampled from the IVC.

Selective venous catheterization

The catheter is advanced along the IVC until the renal vein orifices are entered. Air in the body of the stomach is a fairly good landmark for the level of the renal veins and the only large vein on the left side is the left renal vein. The catheter may sometimes be able to be passed deep into the renal vein, but a guidewire is usually required to position the catheter tip sufficiently distally. Generally it is easier to catheterize the left renal vein first as it is longer than the right renal vein. If the catheter is rotated alternately clockwise and anticlockwise about one-half turn as it is advanced, it will follow the guidewire more freely into the renal vein.

Congenital anomalies of the IVC and in particular the left renal vein occur in 2–9% of studies. These result from persistence of the left supracardinal vein and the intersupracardinal anastomoses.

A test injection of contrast medium (Iopamidol, Omnipaque or equivalent) should be made to confirm correct positioning. Films should be taken for documentation of the catheter position if blood samples are taken. A hand injection and digital subtraction angiography (DSA) or a small film camera (70–110 mm) is sufficient for this purpose.

To make a loop the catheter can be turned either in the left renal vein or across the iliac confluence. Withdraw the guidewire proximal to the expected apex of the loop, rotate the catheter on half turn and advance it. It will advance up the IVC and withdraw from the renal vein or left iliac vein. A loop shorter than 5 cm will not work properly as the tip will lie inside the loop (Fig. 11.3). If the loop is formed in the left renal vein the left adrenal vein may be catheterized by the looped catheter just before it exits the left renal vein. The patient is usually able to feel the tip of the catheter if undue force is exerted on the wall of a vein as it is thin.

The looped cobra has a shape such that the left adrenal vein, both spermatic veins and also the right renal veins may be entered if required. The tip of the catheter is positioned at the vein outlet and the catheter advanced down the vein by gently withdrawing the main catheter shaft. Generally the cathe-

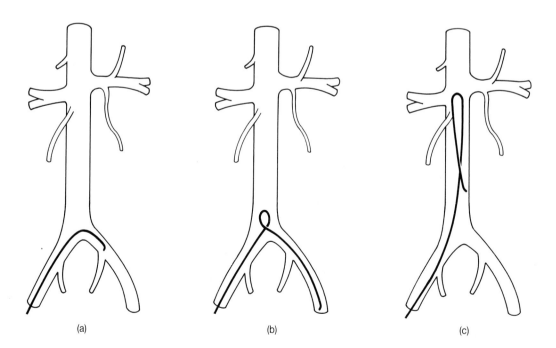

Fig. 11.3 Making a loop in a cobra catheter in the venous system.
(a) The catheter is passed over a guidewire across the iliac venous confluence and down the contralateral external iliac vein for about 6–7 cm.
(b) The guidewire is withdrawn to the iliac confluence and the catheter is twisted one half turn. (c) The catheter is advanced up the inferior vena cava to form a recurved loop rather like a very long Simmon's shape. If the loop is too short the tip of the catheter will curl up on itself.

ter tip needs to be in the vein only a short distance for sampling and deep insertion of the catheter may cause venospasm or wedging of the catheter and inability to aspirate blood. Adrenal vein perforation may cause infarction of the gland from venous thrombosis.

Normally the right adrenal vein arises near the level of the twelfth thoracic vertebra about 3–4 cm above the right renal vein. The right adrenal vein may be quite difficult to catheterize, as the trunk is very short and often many small hepatic veins enter the IVC near the adrenal vein or drain into it. It is important to be sure when sampling that it is from the adrenal gland and not the liver or IVC. Sometimes a double renal curve catheter is more suited for the right adrenal vein than a cobra catheter.

Catheterization of the gonadal veins is usually as a precursor to embolization for varicocele. Either a looped cobra or a Simmons catheter is suitable (Cook; NB5.0–35–100–M–NS–SIM3). The cobra can be advanced further down the vein as the Simmons penetration is limited by the length of the recurved tip. Deflecting guidewires [Cook; TDH 100 (handle), Cook, TDW–28–100–5 (guidewire)] may be used to make a curve in a catheter or to advance a catheter into a vein which has an acute angle with the IVC, but the tip of the deflecting wire must not extend beyond the catheter tip and care should be taken to avoid perforation of a vein.

Some clinicians request simultaneous sampling from each side in which case each renal or adrenal vein should be catheterized and samples obtained at the same time. In most cases samples obtained within a minute or so are quite satisfactory and only a single catheter is required. The only exception is sampling for adrenal corticotrophin hormone (ACTH) which must be performed simultaneously from the right and left petrosal sinuses as the levels of the hormone vary considerably from minute to minute. Although ATCH sampling is not strictly genitourinary, the target organs are, hence its inclusion here. The internal jugular veins on each side are catheterized using a cerebral catheter (Cook; BPS 6.5–5.0–38–100–M–NS–DAV–1) from the femoral vein and a 2.6 Fr coaxial catheter (Cook Explorer) passed along the petrosal vein to the cavernous sinus using a steerable 0.014 inch guidewire (Cook).

Renal venography

Catheter: Cobra 2 catheter (artery) (Cook; HBP5.5–38–80–M–NS–C2)
            Straight catheter with side holes (vein) (Cook; HN5.0–35–65–M–10S–0)
Contrast: Iopromide (Schering AG) or equivalent 300 mgI/ml for DSA : 20–25 ml at 15 ml/sec
            370 mgI/ml conventional films :20–25 ml at 15 ml/sec
Film sequence: 2 per sec for 3 sec
                1 per sec for 4 sec

Catheterize the renal artery with the cobra 2 catheter. Make a 2 cm radius curve in the end of the straight catheter after softening the tip in hot water. Insert the catheter as far into the renal vein as possible. Almost always, the catheter will enter the lower pole veins. Ensure that the tip of the catheter is not wedged and that injected contrast medium flows away freely. Position the patient for the venography and connect the power injector to the venous catheter. Inject 5–8 μg adrenalin slowly into the arterial catheter and wait about 15–20 sec before injecting contrast medium and making the film run.

Warn the patient that they may experience mild discomfort as the injection is made (sometimes a small extravasation occurs) and explain that the adrenaline may make them feel mildly anxious. If branch renal vein thrombosis is suspected, the procedure will need repeating in the upper and possibly the middle portion of the kidney. The use of a steerable guidewire, for example, Terumo glide wire is helpful to reposition the venous catheter.

It is important that the position of the catheter and injection of contrast medium is such that small intrarenal veins will be opacified if patent, as thrombosis at this level can result in the clinical condition of renal vein thrombosis (Fig. 11.4)

The patient's pulse and blood pressure should be checked before and after adrenaline injection. No more than two doses should be given in 30 min and this procedure should be performed with great care in the elderly or in patients with cardiac disease. If renin samples are to be taken at the same time, these must be taken before any adrenaline is injected.

Abort the procedure if a significant extravasation of contrast medium occurs in either kidney.

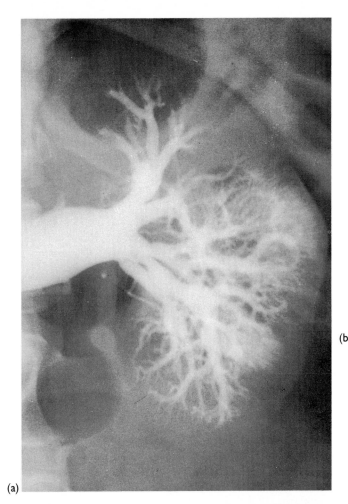

(a)

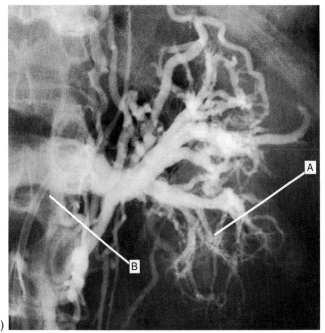

(b)

Fig. 11.4 Renal venography
(a) Normal adrenaline enhanced venogram. The renal veins are well filled with opacification of the intralobular veins and the arcuate veins. The valve at the orifice of the left gonadal vein is patent and the gonadal vein is not filled. (b) Interlobular venous thrombosis. There is patchy filling of the interlobular veins and the arcuate veins are not filled. Multiple small recanalization channels are seen in the lower pole veins (arrow A). Note the arterial catheter (arrow B). (c) Main renal vein occlusion. In this case the filling defect in the renal vein is caused by an unsuspected renal carcinoma extending into the left renal vein and inferior vena cava. Renal venography for major renal vein occlusion has been largely replaced by duplex Doppler ultrasound.

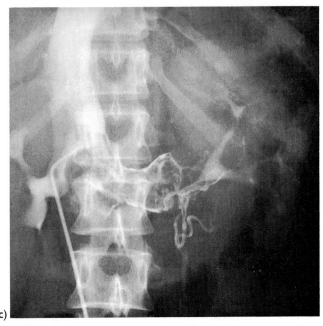

(c)

Renal vein renin sampling

Catheter: Cobra 2 catheter with one side hole
Contrast: Iopromide (Schering AG) or equivalent 300 mgl/ml hand injection of 3–5 ml
Film sequence: 2 per sec for 2 sec

Before embarking on renal vein sampling, it is imperative that you check with the assaying laboratory and referring clinician what is required. You must know how much blood is needed for each sample, what container to put it in, how to store it (often storage on ice is required) and where and when samples are to be taken. Usually two samples are needed from each renal vein and a single sample from the IVC.

Many clinicians require simultaneous samples from the renal veins. This needs two catheters, the second inserted into the contralateral femoral vein or ipsilateral side just inferior to the first catheter. It may be helpful to mark one catheter with sterile tape so there is no confusion regarding which side each catheter is in. Test injections should be performed into each vein and films taken to document correct positioning. This can be done with a hand injection and DSA or camera films taken. Write the order of the samples on the X-ray card and record which samples were taken in the written report.

Adrenal vein sampling and venography

Catheter: Cobra 2 or Spinal catheter (Cook; HBP5.5–38–100–M–NS–HS1)
Contrast: Iopromide (Schering AG) or equivalent 300 mgI/ml
Film sequence: 2 per sec for 3 sec
              1 per sec for 4 sec

It is mandatory to check with the laboratory what samples are needed. Samples are taken from the IVC above and below the adrenal veins and from both renal veins. The tip of the left adrenal catheter should be beyond the entrance of the inferior phrenic vein. It is usually easy to obtain a sample from the left adrenal vein, but it is often difficult to locate the right adrenal vein and even when found and the catheter correctly positioned, it may not be possible to aspi-

rate a sample. If all the other samples are taken as listed above, a rough estimate of the level of activity can be inferred.

Venography alone is hardly ever indicated because of the improvements in CT and ultrasound (US). It is sometimes still requested to confirm the presence of a mass (Fig. 11.5). Complications include adrenal infarction and venous rupture in up to 5–10% of patients. This is more common on the right side.

Testicular vein sampling and venography

Catheter: Cobra 2 (Cook; HBP5.5–38–80–M–NS–C2)
              Simmons (Cook; NB5.0–38–100–M–NS–SIM3)
Contrast: Iopromide (Schering AG) or equivalent 300 mgI$_2$/ml:10–15 ml at 5 ml/sec
Film sequence: 2 per sec for 3 sec
              1 per sec for 4 sec

Venography is indicated in the investigation of a varicocoele and cryptorchidism. The veins are catheterized with a cobra 2 catheter and to pass down the vein, a glide wire (Terumo RF★GA35153) is needed. With varicocoele, which are more com-

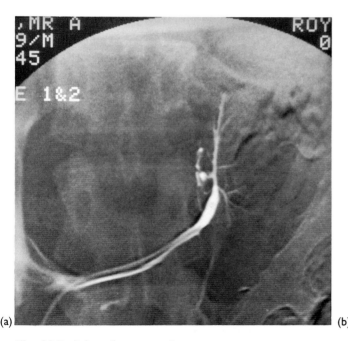

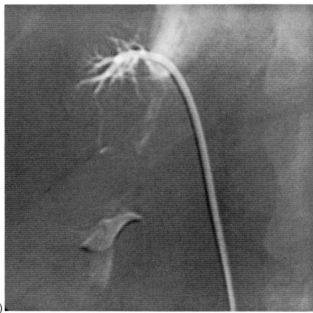

Fig. 11.5 Adrenal venography.
(a) Normal left adrenal venogram with a looped cobra catheter. The tip of the catheter has been placed beyond the entrance of the adrenal outflow. (b) Right adrenal venography. The main portion of the gland is elevated by a metastasis in the lower portion. Cortisol levels in this sample were normal confirming the correct siting of the catheter.

monly left sided and associated with the pelvic congestion syndrome, an injection near the IVC or left renal vein demonstrates the competence of the valves within the vein. Venous sampling looking for the site of abnormal hormone production is indicated in the investigation of masculinization syndromes where the ovary may be the site of production.

Pelvic venography

Catheter: Straight catheter with side holes
Contrast: Iopromide (Schering AG) or equivalent
300 mgl/ml for DSA : 20–25 ml at 15 ml/ sec
370 mgl/ml conventional films : 20– 25 ml at at 15 ml/sec
Film sequence: 2 per sec for 3 sec
1 per sec for 4 sec

Pelvic venography to identify the anatomy of the branches of the internal iliac vein is rarely indicated as it is almost impossible to fill the pelvic veins adequately. Injection of both external iliac veins simultaneously while the patient performs a vigorous Valsalva manouevre will cause reflux of contrast medium into the proximal portion of the internal iliac veins. This has been useful in excluding venous obstruction in the major veins, but is of little value in the diagnosis of pelvic vein thrombosis.

SUGGESTED FURTHER READING

CHERMET J, BIGOT JM (1980) Congenital anomalies of the inferior vena cava. In: *Venography of the Inferior Vena Cava and its Bbranches.* pp. 17–36. Springer-Verlag, Berlin.
KAHN PC (1971) Adrenal venography. In: *Angiography,* second edition. pp. 941–50. Edited by Abrams HL, Little Brown & Company, Boston.

Lasers in urology

Graham Watson

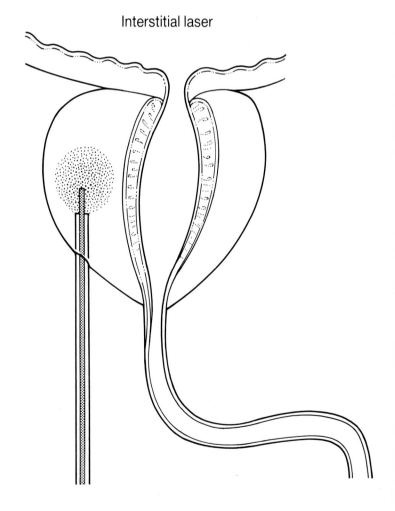

Interstitial laser

INTRODUCTION

Laser energy is a form of intense light energy that has a collimated beam of single wavelength. Following the introduction of lasers for clinical use in the 1960s, applications in urology soon followed. The first clinical application used a ruby laser in the treatment of carcinoma of the penis. Its action on the tumour was found to be enhanced by first coating the penis with a layer of black boot polish. Many varieties of laser are now available with a range of wavelengths from the ultraviolet through the visible spectrum to the infrared. They either deliver a continuous emission of energy (continuous wave) or are pulsed. Being a form of light energy, laser only has an effect when absorbed. The effect of the laser varies according to the wavelength and pulse characteristics used, thus the action of one type of laser energy differs enormously from another, for example, an argon fluoride excimer emits pulses of light in the ultraviolet region and can be used to sculpt a cornea, but is not effective at coagulation. The continuous wave neodymium YAG laser emits a wavelength of 1064 nm, which is near the infrared region. This wavelength is well transmitted by quartz and can therefore be delivered through a fibre. The wavelength is relatively poorly absorbed by tissue and so penetrates deeply, i.e. it has a long pathlength. This causes coagulation. The variety of lasers has sporadically produced some applications where the laser has unique properties.

Until recently, lasers in urology have been an expensive modality, awkward to use with little provable benefit over more traditional treatment options, but this situation has recently changed. Important applications have been developed where lasers may prove to have significant advantages and a new generation of semiconductor lasers adapted from the leisure industry have resulted in highly compact and potentially cheap lasers.

LASER APPLICATIONS IN UROLOGY

Lasers for ureteric stone disease

As a result of research by the author at the Massachusett's General Hospital, a pulsed dye laser was developed for stone fragmentation, the Candela pulsed dye laser (Candela Corporation, Wayland, Massachusetts, USA). This is safer to use than electrohydraulic or ultrasonic lithotripsy because the laser is selectively absorbed by the stone, rather than the tissue around it, eradicating the risk of thermal damage. Miniaturized endoscopes of 7.2 Fr have been introduced because the laser fibre is only 0.25 mm in diameter and this has reduced the complications of ureteroscopy dramatically. For conventional ureteroscopes, a stricture rate of 3% and perforation rate of 7% can be expected at ureteroscopy. With miniaturized scopes, this has fallen to 0 and 0.5%. Once the stone has been visualised, the laser fibre is placed on it and a series of pulses delivered at an energy above the fragmentation threshold (usually 70 MJ via a 320 μg fibre) until the stone is pulverized. Occasionally, the stone starts to migrate proximally up the ureter during fragmentation. Miniaturized endoscopes can be passed right up into the renal pelvis, so the stone is followed and treated where it lies. For those patients in whom initial basketing of a ureteric stone has resulted in a trapped basket within the ureter, the ureteroscope is passed up the ureter alongside the basket and the stone fragmented within it (Fig. 12.1). In the author's experience, 1500 successful ureteroscopic laser lithotripsy cases have been performed. No case of open uretrolithotomy has needed to be performed since 1988.

When using lasers to fragment stones, there is a characteristic noise produced when the fibre is in contact with the stone. This acoustic signal increases

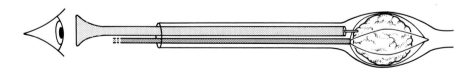

Fig. 12.1 The miniaturized ureteroscope and laser can be passed alongside a basket to fragment the stone trapped within it.

in intensity as the laser energy is increased until fragmentation occurs. No acoustic signal from normal ureter will be heard, but blood clot can mimic stone. Thus, the acoustic signal alone is not sufficient evidence that the laser fibre is in contact with stone. However, it has been found that there is plasma produced when the pulsed dye laser fragments stone. A plasma is a phenomenon produced by high-power flux characterized by ionization, production of white light and noise. The same fibre that delivers the laser energy can transmit this plasma light back to the laser head. By inserting a beam splitter to exclude the primary laser wavelength, the plasma can be looked at alone to identify the stone positively (Fig. 12.2). An alternative system is to look at the light reflected from the target at much lower energies. Using either one of these systems, it is possible to identify positively whether the laser fibre is on stone, tissue or blood clot. The future of minimally invasive techniques is probably gradually to move away from visual control and to use optical feedback systems and external analysis.

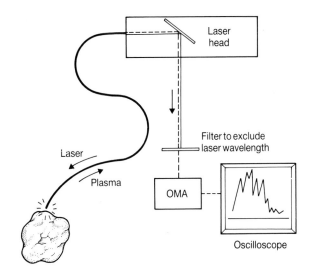

Fig. 12.2 The plasma signal from the laser action on a stone is fed back through the fibre to an optical analyser and displayed on the oscilloscope allowing positive identification.
OMA = optical analyser.

Lasers for bladder tumours

One of the first laser applications in urology was the use of the neodymium YAG laser for coagulating bladder tumours. By using the laser at 40 W for 4 sec, approximately 7 mm of coagulation into the depth of the tumour is achieved. This renders the device only suitable for very small tumours having little advantage over electrocoagulation. In addition, the forward beam of the laser can potentially cause unrecognized bowel injury during treatment.

With the advance of laparoscopic surgery, it is recognized that the bladder can be treated from both surfaces and coagulate tumours, thus minimizing the risk of bowel injury (Fig. 12.3).

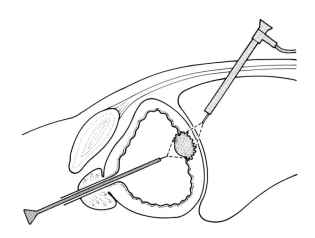

Fig. 12.3 Combined intraluminal and laparoscopic approach to an invasive bladder tumour.

Laser applications for the prostate gland

Although neodymium YAG lasers have been available for 10 years, it is only over the past 2 years that the prostate has come under therapeutic consideration. The average transurethral resection for outflow obstruction is 25 g tissue. The laser is considered too slow a remover of tissue for vapourizing such an amount. Vapourization occurs at temperatures of 200°C and requires a great deal of energy, especially when performed under continuous irrigation, conditions which prevail at cystoscopy. However, it is

now possible to coagulate that amount. Coagulation is a much more efficient use of energy, occurring at temperatures of 60°C. The necrotic tissue will separate from healthy tissue and pass in the urine, the process simulating cryotherapy, which has largely fallen into disrepute because of problems associated with the passage of clot, haemorrhage and infection. The slough produced by laser coagulation is more gelatinous and likened to the mucous seen in ileal conduits.

TRANSURETHRAL LASER-INDUCED PROSTATECTOMY (TULIP)

A neodymium YAG laser at approximately 40 W is delivered at right angles via a prism together with transurethral ultrasound scans at the same sector (Fig. 12.4). A balloon of thermally resistant material which is transparent to laser light is inflated within the prostatic urethra avoiding the distal sphincter and both laser and ultrasound are transmitted through it. A transurethral ultrasound scanner and a prism to deflect the laser beam are introduced centrally within the balloon. The ultrasound scans the prostate at the same level as the laser beam. The prostate from bladder neck to apex is treated under continuous ultrasound control. The whole device is rotated through 90° and the procedure repeated until the whole prostate has been treated. This takes about 20 min and is associated with no bleeding. A suprapubic catheter is left *in situ* until the patient spontaneously voids (usually about 7 days), but the patient is managed as an outpatient.

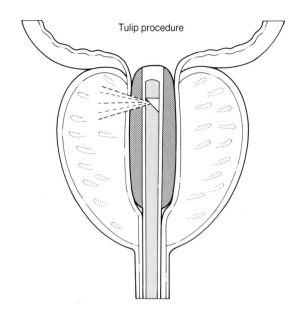

Fig. 12.4 Transurethral laser-induced prostatectomy (TULIP procedure).
A side-firing laser beam moves up and down within the balloon with simultaneous ultrasound scanning.

THE LATERALASE PROCEDURE

This is conceptually identical to the TULIP device, but laser energy is delivered under continuous endoscopic control (Fig. 12.5). Each quadrant of the prostate is treated for 1 min at 60 W. The patient takes several days to re-establish micturition, but the procedure is bloodless and can be done on an outpatient basis.

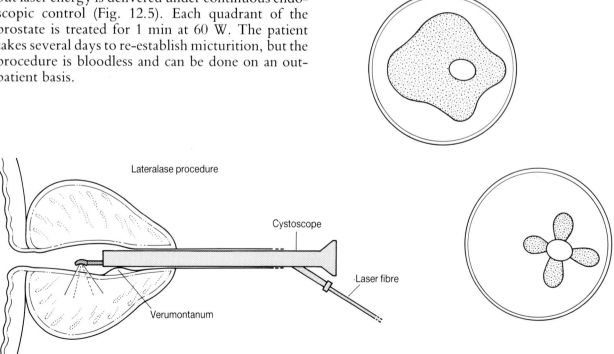

Fig. 12.5 Lateralase procedure.
(a) A device delivering a side-firing beam of laser energy is used to coagulate the prostate under cystoscopic control. (b) A zone of coagulative necrosis coalesces with it's neighbours when sufficient energy is delivered. This sloughs, leaving a cavity.

INTERSTITIAL LASER COAGULATION

Instead of coagulating the prostate from the urethra, the laser is passed perineally into the substance of the prostate (Fig. 12.6). The concept is to produce necrosis of prostatic tissue whilst preserving the urethra and sphincter mechanisms. Presumed resorption of the necrosed tissue then reduces prostatic bulk. Single laser fibres passed repeatedly into the different parts of the prostate or multiple lasers, for exmaple, semiconductor lasers, are techniques currently under study.

All these possible applications cause no bleeding, so irrigation is not necessary. They do not incise or resect the bladder neck, so ejaculation will be preserved. However, if the bladder neck is contributing to the obstruction, the primary aim of the treatment may be lost. For these techniques to become accepted, preoperative selection must be rigorous.

Interstitial coagulation of renal tumours

It has been demonstrated that a simple laser fibre inserted into prostate tissue and used at low power acts as a point source and coagulates approximately 1 cm of tissue. Multiple fibre placements cause a much wider necrosis if sited such that the intervening tissue between adjacent fibres is heated from both sources. Large volumes can thus be coagulated. An alternative approach employs a diffuser tip which causes less charring and more optical penetration into the tumour, therefore treating a larger volume. The surgical laser technology (SLT) hyperthermia system takes temperature measurements from close to the diffuser tip to maintain a temperature at the centre of the tumour at a prefixed level, but below that at which charring occurs. Should the temperature rise above the prefixed range, the laser power is switched off until the temperature falls. Using this system at a power of 20 W, the author has heated a tumour of 8 cm diameter so that the centre is at 90° and the periphery of the kidney at 45° (Fig. 12.7).

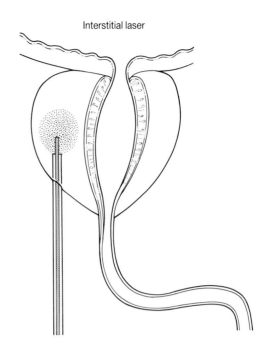

Interstitial laser

Fig. 12.6 Interstitial laser.
A laser fibre can be delivered into the substance of the prostate in order to produce necrosis.

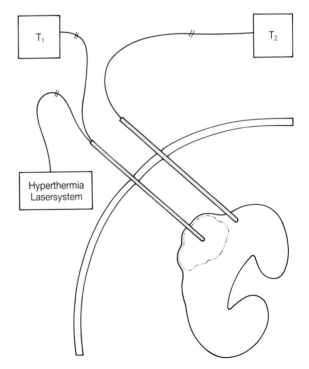

T_1

T_2

Hyperthermia Lasersystem

Fig. 12.7 A laser diffuser is inserted into the centre of the tumour percutaneously.
A thermocouple within the diffuser feeds back to the laser (T_1) to maintain the temperature below 100°C. A second thermocouple at the junction with the normal tissue (T_2) is used to control the volume of tissue heated to the therapeutic level.

SUGGESTED FURTHER READING

BHATTA KM, ROSEN DI, WATSON GM, DRETLER SP (1989) Acoustic and plasma guided lasertripsy of urinary calculi. *Journal of Urology* **142**: 433–37.

ROTH RA, ARETZ TH (1990) TULIP: transurethral laser induced prostatectomy under ultrasound guidance. *Journal of Urology* **142**: 285.

WATSON GM, MURRAY S, DRETLER SP, PARRISH JA (1987) The pulsed dye lased for fragmenting urinary calculi. *Journal of Urology* **138**: 195–98.

WATSON GM, WICKHAM JEA (1989) The development of a laser and miniaturised ureteroscope system for ureteric stone management. *World Journal of Urology* **7**: 147–50.

CHAPTER 13

Alternative treatments for urethral and prostate obstruction

Euan Milroy and David Rickards

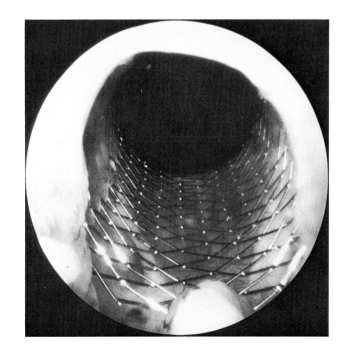

URETHRAL STENTS FOR STRICTURE DISEASE

The many problems with currently available treatments for urethral stricture are well known. Urethral dilation with bougies or balloons and endoscopic urethrotomy cure a few cases, but many recur and with each subsequent treatment more fibrosis at the stricture site increases the risk of later complications. Surgical reconstructive urethroplasty produces excellent results for traumatic strictures, but is less successful for the more common infective or iatrogenic stricture. It was in this clinical context that alternative therapies were sought.

The Urolume™ Wallstent^R (American Medical Systems, Minnesota, USA) was originally designed for endovascular use where it has been successfully used for the prevention of restenosis following angioplasty. It was first implanted into the urethra in 1987.

THE UROLUME WALLSTENT AND DELIVERY TECHNIQUES

The stent is a woven tubular mesh of fine surgical grade superalloy manufactured in various lengths and diameters (Fig. 13.1). Most stents used for urethral stricture have an unconstrained diameter of 14 mm (42 Fr). This is large enough to permit subsequent endoscopy and transurethral bladder surgery. When expanded from its delivery system, it is stable though flexible. It can be deployed in two ways:

1 Catheter-based delivery. This original system was developed for endovascular use. The stent is held in its elongated form under a doubled over plastic membrane on a 9 Fr catheter. When the membrane is pressurized to 3 atm, it peels back allowing the stent to resume its unconstrained diameter. A guidewire is passed into the bladder and the catheter positioned under radiological control at the strictured area and then deployed. Once 50% of the stent has been deployed, it cannot be removed from the urethra without instrumentation and cannot be used again.

2 Endoscopic-based delivery. This permits placement of the stent under direct vision and is the system of choice (Fig. 13.2). A standard 0⁰ telescope is passed down a disposable and sterile device which holds the stent. This consists of an outer moveable sheath which holds the stent in place (Fig. 13.3). The sheath can be retracted allowing the stent to deploy and two safety locks have to be released before the stent is finally released. When it is thought that the stent is in the right position, the telescope is passed through the stent to check is exact position (Figs. 13.4 and 13.5). Should this be wrong, the stent can be pulled back inside the sheath and repositioned as long as the two safety locks have not been released.

Following radiological assessment of the stricture and of its relationship to the sphincters, the stricture is first treated with dilation using bougies or triradiate optical urethrotomy to a 30 Fr under general anaesthesia. The length of the stricture is measured with a calibrated catheter and compared to measurements on the preoperative urethrogram. Once the stent is positioned, no catheter is inserted and should the patient have difficulty in voiding, suprapubic catheter drainage is performed. This prevents damage to the stent before it is covered with epithelium.

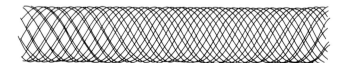

Fig. 13.1 Urolume™ Wallstent^R endoprosthesis.

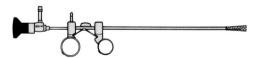

Fig. 13.2 Endoscopic delivery system for implanting the Urolume™ stent.

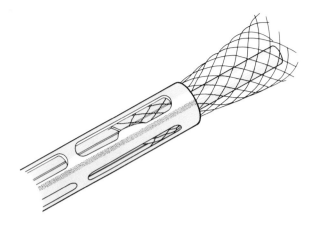

Fig. 13.3 Close up of the stent delivery system.

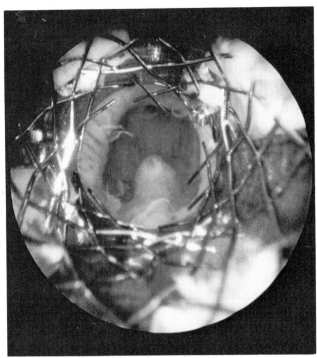

Fig. 13.4 Endoscopic view of the stent and urethra through the delivery system.

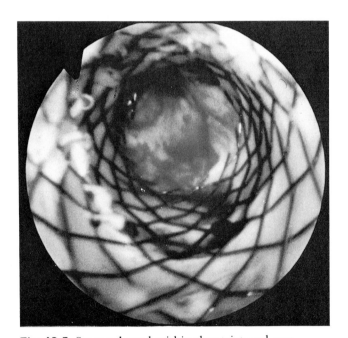

Fig. 13.5 Stent released within the strictured area.

INDICATIONS

The stent is ideally suited for short strictures of the bulbar urethra of any aetiology other than traumatic rupture, although care must be taken in patients following failed urethroplasty procedures. In 50% of these patients, the stent has failed because of a growth of fibrous tissue within the stent lumen presumably because the lining of the urethra is composed of squamous rather than transitional or columnar epithelium. If the intrastent fibrosis causes obstruction, it is incised using an optical urethrotome and a limited resection of the fibrosed tissue is carried out. This usually allows the fibrosed tissue to stabilize with a reasonable intrastent lumen. The stent can be used for sphincter strictures following transurethral surgery or catheterization. If the bladder neck has been damaged by these procedures, significant urinary incontinence is likely which we have subsequently treated successfully with the implantation of an artificial sphincter.

Until more long-term follow-up is available, it is advisable to limit the use of the stent to strictures which have recurred following treatment by at least one or perhaps two urethrotomies or dilations. It would also be advisable not to use the stent in patients younger than 30 years. Strictures near to or involving the distal urethral sphincter mechanism should also be avoided unless the use of an artificial sphincter is envisaged. It is unwise to implant a metallic stent into a severely infected stricture. Strictures up to 4 cm long are suitable.

In the spinal injury patient with detrusor sphincter dyssynergia, the results of endoscopic sphincterotomy are unpredictable. The stent can be used as an alternative in patients with high cervical injuries causing tetraplegia and dyssynergia who have high-pressure voiding unsuitable for intermittent catheterization. Thirteen patients have been treated, four of whom had previously undergone unsuccessful endoscopic sphincterotomy. The stent is positioned across the distal sphincter without initial dilation. At follow-up, all patients were found to be voiding with lower pressures and if not voiding to completion, were leaving smaller residuals.

RESULTS

The stent has now been used in a number of centres in over 300 patients with urethral strictures and with follow-up for up to 4 years. The stent is ideally suitable for bulbar stricture and results have been very good (Fig. 13.6a–b). Many patients get a minor degree of discomfort in the perineum for up to 2 weeks. If the stent is inserted too far downstream in the penile urethra, pain will be experienced with erections, but in the patients we have treated with this problem, pain has resolved spontaneously within 3 months. A number of patients suffer some post micturition dribbling and incontinence of urine for the first 3–6 months. In most, this resolves spontaneously and is due to an inflammatory exu-

date from the reactive epithelial tissue seen during stent healing (Fig. 13.7a and b). In a few, it is because some urine is held within the lumen of the stent at the end of micturition which, with movement, gradually empties.

OTHER URETHRAL STENTS

One other permanent stent has been used for urethral strictures. This is the titanium mesh ASI stent initially designed for use in the prostatic urethra and is fully described below.

Yachia (1990) has described a temporarily implanted urethral stent (Urocoil[R]). This is a spiral coil of stainless steel which is left in a previously dilated urethral stricture for a period of months to allow epithelial covering outside the stent which is then removed endoscopically. It is difficult to see what will prevent strictures recurring after removal of the coil.

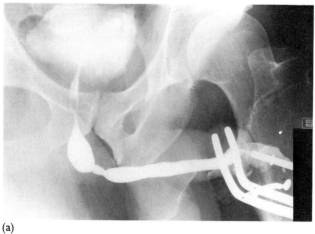

(a)

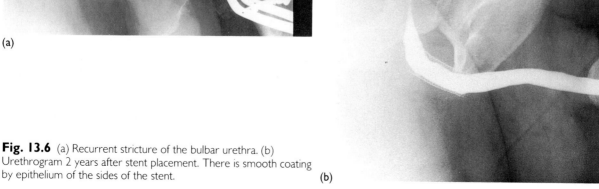

(b)

Fig. 13.6 (a) Recurrent stricture of the bulbar urethra. (b) Urethrogram 2 years after stent placement. There is smooth coating by epithelium of the sides of the stent.

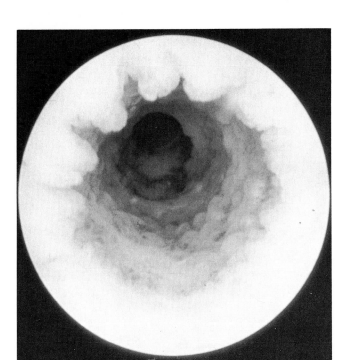
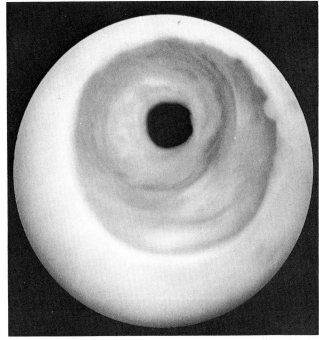

Fig. 13.7 (a) Endoscopic view of hyperplasia 2 months after stent insertion. (b) At 9 months, the urethra is smooth, the stent fully covered by epithelium.

PROSTATE STENTS

Anxiety about the risks of performing prostate surgery on elderly or unfit patients has generated considerable interest in a variety of devices for mechanically holding open the prostatic urethra without the need for major surgery. Stents for temporary and permanent use are now available.

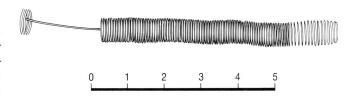

Fig. 13.8 Urospiral prostate stent.

TEMPORARY PROSTATE STENTS

Fabian (1980) first described an indwelling urethral device to replace a permanent urethral catheter for the treatment of prostate obstruction. It consists of a closely coiled spiral of stainless steel wire, narrow at its inner end to allow for its insertion into the urethra. At the outer end, a single wire extends across the distal sphincter and is contiguous with another smaller coil. This stabilizes the coil within the prostatic urethra. The stent will encrust if left too long and will not epithelialize. Cystoscopy cannot be performed whilst the stent is in position, but can be easily removed. It works well as a temporary device and is marketed by Porges as the Urospiral (Fig. 13.8).

A modification of the Urospiral by a Danish company (Engineers and Doctors) involves gold plating the device to reduce the rate of encrustation (Fig. 13.9) and is marketed as the Prostakath. Encrustation will still occur if the stent is left in for too long, but good results have been reported in patients with acute urinary retention unfit for surgery.

Both the Urospiral and the Prostakath are made in various lengths. The diameter of each device is fixed and there is no intrinsic means of fixing the stent within the prostatic urethra. Some stents migrate

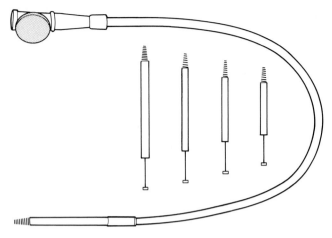

Fig. 13.9 Prostakath prostate stent and introducer.

PERMANENT PROSTATE STENTS

Two stents are available. They are the American Medical Systems Urolume™ Wallstent[R] and the Advanced Surgical Intervention (ASI) titanium mesh stent.

THE UROLUME WALLSTENT AND DELIVERY TECHNIQUES

Catheter-based delivery

Our early experience in 17 patients was with the catheter-based delivery system (Fig. 13.11). The stent was positioned within the prostate cavity and the radial forces exerted by the mesh of the stent held it in position, preventing any possibility of displacement and allowing urothelium to grow over the implanted material. Under local anaesthesia, the patient lies in the left lateral position and a careful urethroscopy is performed with a flexible cystoscope. Transrectal ultrasound using a linear array probe giving a sagittal section of the prostate is then performed to measure prostate length from the bladder neck to the verumontanum (as identified by flexible cystoscopy). A guidewire is inserted through the urethra into the bladder and the Urolume stent on its catheter inserted over the guidewire into the bladder. The compressing doubled over membrane is pressurized to 3 atm with

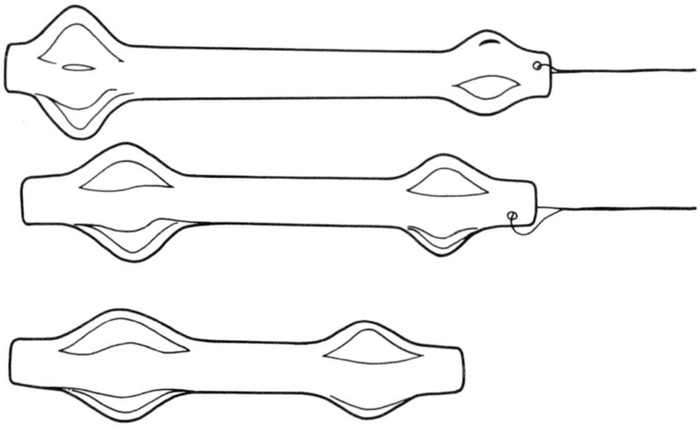

proximally into the bladder or distally into the sphincter mechanism. They can be inserted under radiological or transrectal ultrasound guidance or under direct endoscopic vision under local anaesthesia, an advantage in this group of patients.

Nissenkorn (1989) has described a urethral stent which consists of a short double Malecot 16 Fr polyurethane catheter (Fig. 13.10). The short length of the catheter lies in the prostatic urethra with the inner Malecot at the bladder neck and the outer end of the catheter with it's retention device lying at the verumontanum. The catheter is available in 45, 55 and 60 mm lengths and can be inserted through a cystoscope sheath under transrectal ultrasound or cystoscopic control. A nylon suture is threaded through the distal end of the device and emerges from the urethra to facilitate the stent's removal. The device can only be left *in situ* for 18 weeks without complication and is marketed by Angiomed.

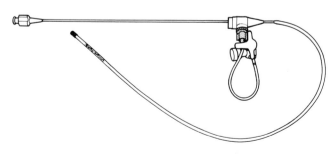

Fig. 13.10 Nissenkorn prostate catheter.

Fig. 13.11 Original catheter mounted delivery system for Wallstent[R].

normal saline allowing the outer membrane to peel back to open one-third of the stent. The whole device is then gently withdrawn under ultrasound guidance until the inner margin of the partially open stent lies exactly at the bladder neck. The membrane can then be fully withdrawn deploying the stent fully into the prostatic urethra. Fourteen millimetre (42 Fr) diameter stents of varying lengths (20–30 mm) are used and if the prostate length exceeds this, overlapping stents can be inserted. The position of the stent is checked by flexible cystoscopy. Occasionally, the stent fails to expand fully. In these cases, a 12 mm by 4 cm balloon is inserted and inflated within the stent.

In all our 17 patients, the stent held open the prostatic urethra and distal sphincter function (upon which urinary continence solely depended) was not impaired. However, exact positioning at the bladder neck proved difficult and at follow-up cystoscopy, free wires uncovered by urothelium were seen protruding into the bladder in seven patients. This precipitates encrustation and stone formation. It remains a useful technique for patients whose immobility or other medical conditions prevent them from lying in lithotomy, the position necessary for the endoscopic delivery system.

Endoscopic delivery

With the patient in lithotomy position and under local anaesthesia, prostate length is measured by transrectal ultrasound and cystoscopy. The device holding the stent is then inserted and the stent deployed at the bladder neck under direct vision, using a 0^0 telescope. Before the safety lock is released which permits final deployment of the stent, the stent position is checked by moving the telescope along the full length of the device within the prostatic urethra. The verumontanum and the position of the distal sphincter mechanism can be seen through slots. If the stent position is not correct, the device is retracted enclosing the stent within the sheath permitting repositioning. The inner end of the stent should lie exactly at the bladder neck and the outer end should fully cover the lateral lobes of the prostate. Once the position is observed to be correct, the safety lock is released allowing the stent to assume its final position (Fig. 13.13).

Eighty patients have been treated in this way, the majority presenting with acute or chronic retention. Following insertion, most patients suffer frequency, urgency and occasional incontinence, but as epithelium covers the stent (Fig. 13.12), these symp-

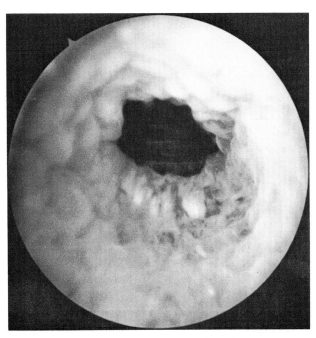

Fig. 13.12 Endoscopic appearance of Urolume prostate stent at 9 months. Complete covering with epithelium.

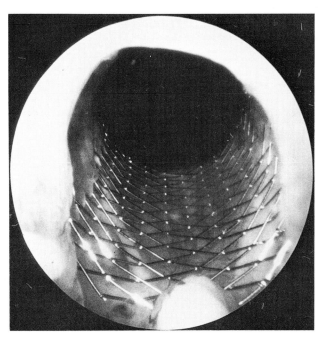

Fig. 13.13 Endoscopic appearance of prostate Urolume™ Wallstent^R immediately after deployment.

toms settle within 1–2 months. 2 % stents have had to be removed, four because of poor positioning within the prostatic urethra, two causing incontinence. One stent was removed at 11 months at the patient's request because of severe and persistent detrusor instability. The epithelium covering the stent was resected endoscopically, the stent pushed into the bladder and then removed.

The Advanced Surgical Intervention Inc. stent

The Advanced Surgical Intervention (ASI) (San Clemente California) stent is the only other stent available for the permanent treatment of prostate obstruction. The stent is made of titanium fixed mesh loaded onto a prostate balloon dilation catheter and positioned under fluoroscopic, ultrasound or direct endoscopic vision control. The 12 mm stent is mounted over the balloon, which when inflated forces open the titanium mesh into the prostate. The ASI stent (Fig. 13.14) works well in clinical trials and in patients with acute retention and early results confirm that it is covered by epithelium.

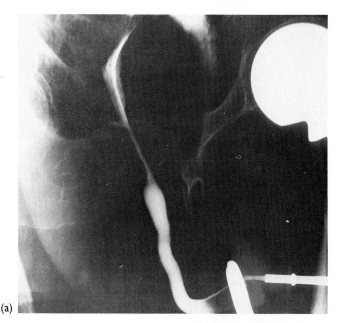

(a)

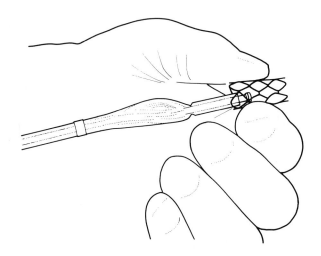

Fig. 13.14 Advanced Surgical Intervention balloon mounted prostate stent, fully expanded.

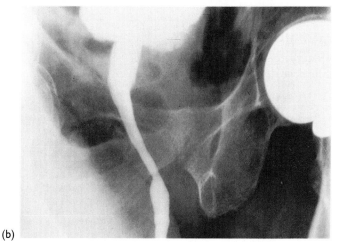

(b)

Fig. 13.15 (a) Urethrogram of unfit patient with acute retention. (b) Same patient voiding normally after insertion of Urolume™ prostate stent.

Indications for stent insertion

In the elderly or unfit patient for whom prostate surgery would be a risk and in whom pharmacological treatment might cause unacceptable side effects, some form of prostate stenting to relieve acute retention or severe prostatic symptoms offers an excellent alternative, providing it can be performed under local anaesthesia and rapidly (Fig. 13.15 a and b).

Balloon dilation of the prostatic urethra

The theory that by dilating an obstructed prostate gland will relieve symptoms of outflow obstruction is not new. Metal dilators, bougies and the human finger have all been used for this purpose, but they have not gained wide acceptance over transurethral surgery. New balloon technology has revived dilation as an alternative to surgery and it has certain appeals, the major being preservation of fertilty because the bladder neck is not rendered incompetent.

Technique

The procedure is performed under local anaesthetic and antibiotic cover with the patient upon a fluoroscopy table in the supine–oblique position. Culture of the urine before the procedure is performed to ensure there is no infection present. A retrograde urethrogram using a Knutson's clamp is performed to assess the position of the distal sphincter mechanism, length of the prostatic urethra and position of the bladder neck. The position of the distal sphincter is marked by either reference to an underlying bony structure of by positioning a fine needle percutaneously at the level of the sphincter. A straight guidewire is then inserted through the urethra into the bladder. The balloon dilation catheter is passed over the guidewire and positioned within the prostatic urethra in such a way that the distal sphincter and bladder neck are not included within the length of the balloon. The position of the balloon can be checked by passing a small infant feeding catheter alongside the balloon up the anterior urethra and injecting a small amount of contrast medium. The balloon is then gently inflated and traction applied to the catheter as during inflation the balloon tends to migrate into the bladder. During inflation, the patient is likely to experience considerable perineal pain and urgency. The balloon should be left inflated for 10 min (Fig. 13.16), deflated and then removed. The bladder needs to be irrigated with saline because the procedure produces much bleeding and a urethral catheter left in place for 24 hours. This can then be removed as long as the patient spontaneously micturates.

Complications

1 Haematuria. This is rarely prolonged and usually settles with conservative therapy, mainly urethral catheterization.
2 Acute urinary retention. This is more likely to occur in patients with very large benign hyperplasias of the prostate.
3 Infection. Prostatic and seminal vesicle inflammatory disease may be expected in some patients and is more likely to occur in those with a pre-existing urinary tract infection.
4 Incontinence. As with any intervention to the prostate gland, relief of obstruction may unmask detrusor instability which then results in urge incontinence. Incontinence may also be due to damage to the distal sphincter mechanism. This serious complication must be avoided by correct placement of the balloon catheter. Lower tract urodynamics will be needed to differentiate the cause of obstruction.

Indications

Balloon dilation is suitable for those patients with a moderate degree of benign prostatic hyperplasia in whom there is not inappropriate enlargement of the central zone of the gland superiorly (what used to be referred to as the middle lobe). No such lobe exists in McNeal's classification of the prostate's zonal anatomy). This configuration of prostate enlargement can be clearly identified on suprapubic vesical ultrasound or with forward-looking probes with transrectal ultrasound. Other contraindications of balloon dilation are:

1 Carcinoma of the prostate
2 Urethral stricture
3 Bladder neck obstruction or dyssynergia
4 Chronic prostatic inflammatory disease
5 Bladder carcinoma
6 Bladder stones

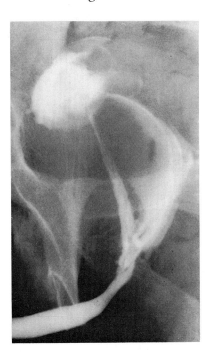

Fig. 13.16 Balloon dilation of the prostate.
The balloon has been inflated within the prostatic urethra leaving the distal sphincter mechanism and the bladder neck intact.

Results

It is claimed that 70–85% of patients gain symptomaic relief and that 60% improve urodynamically. Despite this procedure being easy to perform with a low morbidity and a low cost factor, it has not gained general acceptance, because of poor long term results.

REFERENCES

FABIAN KM (1980) Der intraprostatische 'Partielle Katheter' (Urologische Spirrle). *Urologe* **194**: 236–238.

NISSENKORN I (1990) A new self retaining intraurethral device. *Brit J Urology*, **65**: 197–200.

YACHIA D, CASK D and ROBINSON S (1990) Self retaining intraurethral stent: an alternative to long term indwelling catheter or surgery in the treatment of prostatism. *Am J Radiology* **154**: 111–13.

Suggested further reading

CHAPPLE CR, MILROY EM, RICKARDS D (1990) Permanently implanted urethral stent for prostatic outflow obstruction in the unfit patient-preliminary report. *British Journal of Urology* **66**: 58–65.

MILROY EM, CHAPPLE CR, COOPER JE (1988) A new treatment for urethral stricture. *Lancet* **1**: 1424–27.

NIELSON KK, KROMANN-ANDERSEN B, NORDLING J (1989) Relationship between detrusor pressure and urinary flow rate in males with an intra-urethral prostatic spiral. *British Journal of Urology* **64**: 275–79.

SHAW PJR, MILROY EJG, TIMONEY AG, ELDIN A, MITCHELL N (1990) Permanent external sphincter stents in spinal injury patients. *British Journal of Urology* **66**: 297–302.

CASTANEDA F, BANNO J, BRADY T (1991) Prostatic urethroplasty with balloon catheter as a nonsurgical alternative to benign prostatic hyperplasia. *Radiological Clinics of North America* **29**: 591–603.

CHAPTER 14

Upper tract urodynamics: The Whitaker test

David Rickards and Jeremy Noble

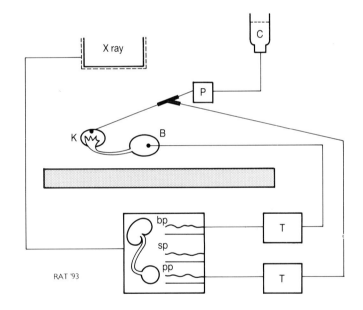

INTRODUCTION

The urinary tract consists of two mutually dependent components: the 'upper tract – kidneys and ureters' and the 'lower tract–bladder and urethra'. The kidney continually produces urine which is stored in the pelvicalyceal system which empties periodically at low pressures, less than 10 cm H_2O. The ureter functions as a distensible conduit with intrinsic peristalsis to transport urine from the pelvi-ureteric junction down through a uni-directional valve at the vesico ureteric junction at pressures up to 60 cm H_2O. The latter mechanism protects the nephrons from damage by the transmission of back pressure. Like the pelvicalyceal system, the bladder stores urine at low pressures and periodically empties at high pressures. The urethra has sphincters to maintain continence and is a distensible conduit. Both sexes have two sphincter mechanisms. The proximal sphincter in the male (bladder neck mechanism) provides a powerful block to the retrograde passage of semen during ejaculation and serves both a genital and urinary role. In the female there is no significant anatomical or functional mechanism at this site. The more distal of the two mechanisms, merging with the distal end of the prostate in the male and encompassing most of the length of the female urethra is the distal sphincter mechanism. Either of these two sphincter mechanisms can by themselves produce urinary continence in the male. Anything that compromises the normal function of the distal sphincter mechanism in the female will result in incontinence. It is therefore not surprising in clinical practice that male patients are likely to suffer from outflow obstruction, whereas females are troubled by incontinence.

Standard radiological investigation provides anatomical information that contributes little to the understanding of function. Current techniques aimed at assessing function are encompassed by the term 'urodynamics', many of which require some form of intervention, whether that be urethral catheterization or percutaneous access to the upper urinary tract. It is vitally important that any tube inserted into a patient for the purposes of obtaining accurate physiological measurements should be correctly sited with the minimum upset to the organ under investigation.

UPPER URINARY TRACT URODYNAMICS

The traditional dogma that 'dilation is synonymous with obstruction' has been proven to be far from accurate and it is now accepted clinical practice that 'dilatation does *not* equal obstruction'. Causes of dilation without obstruction include:

1 High urine flow states
2 Vesicoureteric reflux
3 Urinary diversions
4 Primary megacalyces
5 Ureteric surgery
6 Atonic renal pelvis
7 Postobstruction dilation

The pelvicalyceal system does not normally generate a pressure of more than 15 cm H_2O, but in acute obstruction it can produce pressures as high as 60 cm H_2O which causes ischaemia and potentially irreversible renal damage. Acute obstruction is usually clinically evident, perhaps needing percutaneous nephrostomy to relieve the upper tract of its high pressures. The classic findings on excretory urography of a delayed pyelogram and a persistent dense nephrogram with delayed films to pinpoint the level and perhaps cause of obstruction are well known.

Efficient ureteric peristalsis is dependent upon the ureteric walls being able to oppose. Ureteric dilation, whether obstructive or not, or disorders of wall mobility prevent the ureteric walls opposing, compromising the efficient transport of urine and tubular flow. The normal response of the upper tract to obstruction at or above the vesico–ureteric junction is an increase in the rate of ureteric and pelvic peristalsis and eventual dilation. Dilation causes discoordinated peristalsis and inefficient transport of urine. As flow is reduced down the ureter, pressure rises are first transmitted to the collecting ducts, then along the tubules to the glomeruli. If there is no parallel increase in the glomerular hydrostatic pressure, filtration will eventually stop.

Chronic loin pain and/or deteriorating renal function where an obstructing or functional ureteric lesion has not been excluded or where the significance of an obstructing lesion is in doubt requires more than standard imaging techniques. Diuresis excretory urography has little to offer as the anatomical demonstration of a dilated system neither confirms nor excludes obstruction. Diuresis renography, radionuclide parenchymal transit times and pressure flow studies are the techniques now used to investigate equivocally obstructed kidneys.

Nuclear medicine studies are of particular importance in providing an assessment of differential renal function and are essential in serial follow-up. Doppler ultrasound (US) with the measurement of the resistive index (the result of the peak systolic velocity minus the lowest diastolic velocity divided by the peak systolic velocity) is useful for acute obstruction, but is a difficult measurement to make, not very reproducible and of little use in the evaluation of chronic obstruction. When doubt exists, the Whitaker test is performed.

The steps involved are:

1 Antegrade pyelography or percutaneous nephrostomy
2 Pressure flow studies
3 Documentation of the relevant anatomy

Antegrade pyelography or percutaneous nephrostomy

Upper tract pressure flow studies have to be performed through a needle or catheter placed within the collecting system. This can be achieved by:

1 Performing a standard *antegrade pyelogram* with a 21 gauge needle as described in Chapter 2. This has the advantage of being virtually atraumatic, but the disadvantage of using a single needle for both perfusion and pressure measurements and the danger of the needle migrating out of the collecting system during the study. Also, the study can only be done at one sitting. To repeat it the next day would require another puncture.
2 Performing *percutaneous nephrostomy*. If there is a pre-existing drainage tube within the kidney, the study can be performed through it. Otherwise, the insertion of a nephrostomy tube is an option. The advantages are that there is little chance of extravasation and that the study can be repeated as often as needed. Ambulatory upper tract studies have to be performed through a nephrostomy tube. The disadvantages are that a single channel is being used for both perfusion and pressure changes.
3 Performing a *double puncture*. Either two antegrade needles, two nephrostomy tubes or one of each are inserted into the collecting system. This has the advantage that pressure changes can be recorded through one and perfusion through the other. This provides better pressure traces and more accurate diagnostic information. The disadvantage is that with two punctures, the complication rate is increased.

4 Performing a *single puncture with a double lumen catheter*. This is the most attractive option and many companies are producing such a catheter, but as yet not one that is suitable.

Irrespective of the technique used, it is important that a test injection of contrast medium shows that there is no extravasation.

Pressure-flow studies

Bladder pressure is measured via a urethral catheter connected to a transducer (Fig. 14.1). Renal pelvic pressure can be measured through a nephrostomy tube or through a needle placed in the collecting system at antegrade pyelography. The puncture technique needs to be good as any leak from the collecting system degrades the information that pressure studies will provide. Through one arm of a 'Y' connector, dilute contrast (e.g. Urographin 150, Schering AG, Berlin) is infused at an initial rate of 10 ml/min whilst the other arm of the 'Y' is connected to a pressure transducer recording renal pelvic pressure in response to perfusion. The bladder pressure is continuously recorded and the subtracted pressure (pelvic pressure − bladder pressure) automatically calculated. Such manometric equipment is available

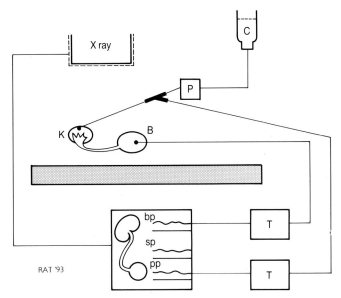

Fig. 14.1 Diagramatic representation of upper urinary tract urodynamics: the Whitaker test.
Contrast (C) is pumped through a 'Y' connector into the kidney (K) at a specific rate (10 ml/min). Pressure changes within the renal pelvis are recorded via a pressure transducer (T) to give total pelvic pressure (pp). The bladder pressure is also recorded (bp). The difference between the total pelvic pressure and the bladder pressure is the subtracted pressure (sp). Synchronous fluoroscopy provides detailed anatomical information. B = bladder.

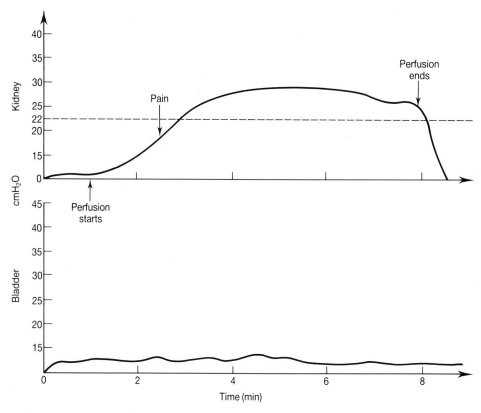

Fig. 14.2 Obstructive upper tract study.
At the start of perfusing the kidney at a rate of 10 ml/min, the renal pelvic pressure rises to above 22 cm H_2O and is associated with loin pain. The bladder pressure during the study remains below 15 cm H_2O and is associated with loin pain. The bladder pressure during the study remains below 15 cm H_2O, normal during filling.

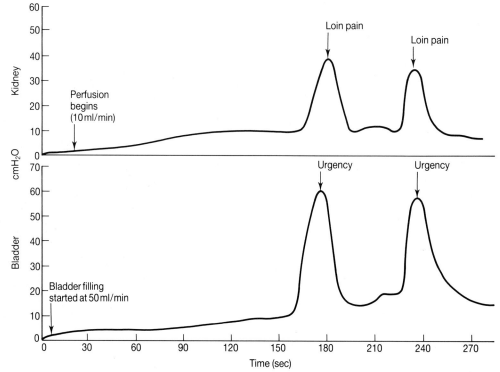

Fig. 14.3 There are unstable contractions of the detrusor (bladder) muscle during filling which produce both loin pain and simultaneous rises in pressure within the renal pelvis. This patient has an unstable bladder and vesicoureteric reflux.

in any department performing lower urinary tract urodynamics. Using this technique a pressure difference between the upper and lower urinary tract of less than 15 cm H_2O excludes obstruction. If the renal pelvic pressure exceeds the bladder pressure by more than 22 cm H_2O, obstruction is confirmed (Fig. 14.2). Pressure differentials between 15 and 22 cm H_2O is an equivocal range. If both the bladder and pelvic pressure rise equally together, vesicoureteric reflux may have occurred (Fig. 14.3) in the presence of high bladder pressures either during filling (unstable detrusor) or during voiding. Higher rates of perfusion have been advocated, but are of debatable clinical usefulness. Perfusion at 10 ml/min is considerably in excess of physiological rates. The effect of bladder filling on upper tract pressures must also be taken into account especially if the patient's symptoms are related to micturition or where vesicoureteric reflux has already been established. Simultaneous perfusion and pressure monitoring of both the upper tracts at 10 ml/min and the bladder at 50 ml/min is performed.

Documentation of relevant anatomy

Simultaneous fluoroscopy defines the anatomy of the upper tract and spot films are taken.

COMPLICATIONS

These are related to the initial puncture of the collecting system and are the same as for antegrade pyelography or percutaneous nephrostomy. If the renal pelvic pressure is allowed to go too high, pyelosinus backflow or forniceal rupture will occur. This may precipitate pain. Infection is always a concern and the procedure should be covered by antibiotics.

SUGGESTED FURTHER READING

FLOWER, CDR (1977) Wide ureters, a dilemma in diagnosis. *British Journal of Radiology* **50**: 539–40.

HOLDEN D, GEORGE NJR, RICKARDS, D, BARNARD RJ, O'RIELLY, PH (1984) Renal pelvic pressures in human chronic obstructive uropathy. *British Journal of Urology* **56**: 565–67.

LUPTON, EW, RICKARDS D, TESTA TJ, GILPIN, SA, GOSLING, JA, BARNARD RJ (1985) A comparison of diuresis renography, the Whitaker test and renal pelvic morphology in idiopathic hydronephrosis. *British Journal of Urology* **57**: 119–23.

PFISTER RC, YODER IL and NEWHOUSE JH (1981) Percutaneous urological procedures. *Seminars in Roentgenology* **16**2: 135–51.

WEINBERG SL (1976) Ureteral function III. *Investigative Urology* **13**: 339.

WHITAKER RH (1973) Methods of assessing obstruction in dilated ureters. *British Journal of Urology* **45**: 15–22.

WHITAKER RH (1982) Pressure flow studies. In: *Idiopathic Hydronephrosis*, pp. 62–7. Edited by O'RIELLY PH, GOSLING JA Springer-Verlag, Berlin Heidelberg, New York.

Impotence: Radiological considerations

Simon J. Hampson, William R. Lees and David Rickards

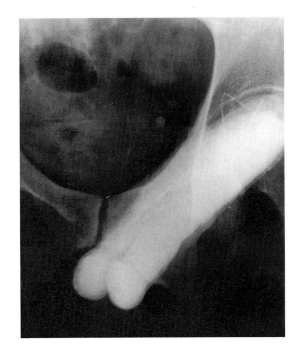

Impotence is a common problem, the exact incidence of which is difficult to define but contemporary evidence from the USA suggests 1 in 10 adult males are affected. Medical and surgical therapies for organic impotence are evolving as is the interest in and technology for diagnosis. Increasing numbers of men are presenting for investigation and treatment.

RELEVANT ANATOMY AND PHYSIOLOGY

The penis consists of three erectile components: the two corpora cavernosa forming the shaft and the ventral corpus spongiosum expanding distally as the glans. The wall of the corpora is a thick fibrous tissue, the tunica albuginea. This contains a mesh of endothelium-lined sinusoids supported in a loose fibromuscular stroma. The corpora cavernosa communicate with each other through a central septum.

Arterial blood reaches the penis via the internal pudendal arteries. After crossing the medial border of the inferior pubic ramus and giving off perineal and scrotal branches these vessels become the penile arteries. These are short trunks which divide to form four branches: (1) the dorsal artery which supplies the glans penis and the penile skin, (2) the urethral artery, (3) the bulbar artery and (4) the cavernosal artery, which is the main source of blood to the erectile tissues of the penis. The latter run through the centre of each corpora giving off numerous helicine arteries which feed into the sinusoids. The terminations of the bulbar and dorsal arteries anastomose with each other in the glans penis.

Venous blood leaving the sinusoids can follow one of several separate routes. The deep drainage system consists of the crural veins which drain into the pudendal venous plexus after leaving the root of the penis. In the proximal third of the penis there is an extensive venous network which forms the cavernosal veins before merging with the internal pudendal veins. Emissary veins also pass directly through the tunica albuginea and run along its surface before joining the deep dorsal vein. This pierces the suspensory ligament of the penis and passes upwards in the midline between the symphysis pubis and the perineal membrane to empty into the periprostatic venous plexus.

Erection is the end result of a complex interplay of psychogenic stimuli, neurogenic impulses and vascular changes within a satisfactory hormonal enviroment. The most active components in this event are the small arteries of the penis and the sinusoids they supply. In the flaccid state there is a basal adrenergic drive resulting in sinusoidal constriction with flow into the corpora occurring only in systole. There is free egress of blood from sinusoids to venules running both within the corpora and also out through the tunica. Once erection is initiated there is relaxation of the arterial and sinusoidal smooth muscle resulting in increased arterial inflow to the corpora. Relaxation of the sinusoids results in compression of the venules against other sinusoids and also the tunica albuginea. The trapping of blood within the corpora goes on until the pressure in the corpora

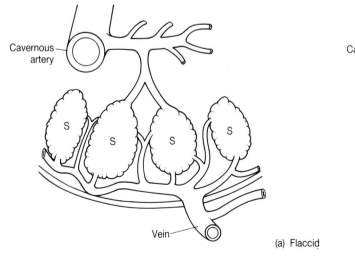

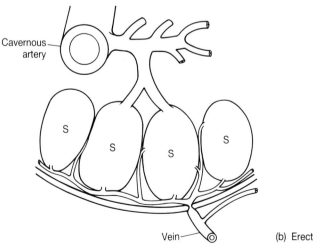

Fig. 15.1 Diagrammatic representation of erect and flaccid penis in transverse section.
(a) In the flaccid state there is smooth muscle constriction within the corpora and easy egress of blood from the cavernosal sinusoids. (b) In the erect state increased blood flow and smooth muscle relaxation compress venules and blood is trapped in the corpora.

approaches the arterial systolic pressure. At full erection there should be minimal flow of blood from the corpora (Fig. 15.1). Detumescence occurs with withdrawal of excitatory stimuli, reflexly with ejaculation and in the presence of high adrenergic drive.

INVESTIGATION

General

Careful history taking should identify the majority of patients with nonorganic impotence. Details should be taken of past medical events or traumatic episodes. Medication and cigarette habit should be altered as far as possible. Physical examination will identify patients with gross anatomical, hormonal, vascular or neurogenic problems. Most patients will undergo blood testing to check blood sugar, testosterone levels, prolactin levels and thyroid function. Clinical evaluation is important; patients with a psychogenic history should have counselling and those who are not prepared to undergo surgery should not have contrast studies. Further investigation should obtain objective evaluation of the penile vasculature and classify the aetiology of the impotence into one of four clinically useful groups:

1 Arterial disease or failure to fill
2 Venous leakage or failure to store
3 A combination of 1) and 2)
4 Normal penile vasculature

Investigative possibilities are many (Table 15.1). Colour Doppler ultrasound and cavernosometry are most widely used. Doppler ultrasound will diagnose whether there is sufficient inflow of arterial blood in response to vasoactive agents for erection, whether

Nocturnal penile tumescence monitoring
Penile–brachial pressure index
Duplex ultrasonography
Colour Doppler imaging
Cavernosometry
Cavernosography
Arteriography
Plethysmography
Radionucleotide studies
Nerve conduction studies

Table 15.1 *Investigative techniques in impotence*

there is a leak of veins or whether there is a possible combination of both arteriogenic and venogenic causes of impotence and should be the first line of investigation. Cavernosometry will document the degree of venous leakage and the anatomy of the draining veins, but is only performed once it is known that there is no arterial insufficiency.

Vasoactive agents

All tests of erectile function can be performed before and after the injection of vasoactive (smooth-muscle relaxant) agents to the corpora. The most commonly used agent is papaverine hydrochloride which can be used in combination with phentolamine. Prostaglandin E1 may be effective when other agents fail. All vasoactive agents carry the risk of priapism and the dose administered to an individual patient should take account of the clinical picture. As a rule we administer 10 mg papaverine for each decade of life.

Injection technique

Vasoactive agents are injected directly into the corpora through a 25G or 21G butterfly needle. If performing colour Doppler ultrasound, the needle is placed in the base of one corpus cavernosum as it is held by the thumb and index finger of the hand (Fig. 15.2). For cavernosometry, a needle is placed just proximal to the glans penis into each corpus cavernosa from the lateral aspect. This will insure that as erection is induced, the needles will not migrate out of the corpus which would precipitate either incorrect pressure readings or extravasation of contrast medium or saline during injection. The tunica will present resistance and a distinct 'give' is felt as this is passed. Tourniquets are not used, but dispersion of the vasoactive agent is improved if the base of the penis is massaged.

Erectile grade

Although there will be subjective variability the quality of the erection obtained after injection of the vasoactive agent should be graded:

Grade 0 = no response
Grade 1 = tumescence but no deviation from the vertical
Grade 2 = tumescence but less than 90° deviation
Grade 3 = normal response, suitable for penetration

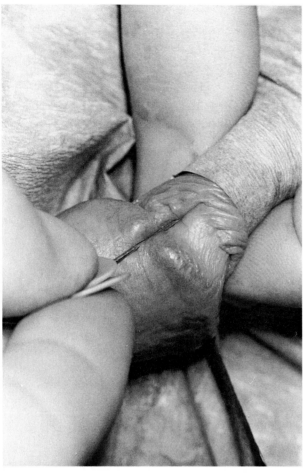

Fig. 15.2 One corpora is held firmly at the base of the penis.

A 23G needle (in this case a butterfly) is passed through the tunica albuginea. There is a distinct 'give' as this happens. If doubt remains imaging should be used to confirm intracorporeal placement.

Colour Doppler imaging

Colour Doppler imaging (Acuson 128 XP, Mountain View, California) is capable of visualizing blood flow over the entire field of the ultrasound image and encoding the blood flow velocity pixel by pixel according to a colour scale. It can document the number of cavernosal arteries, their tortuosity and the presence of abnormal collateral vessels. Colour Doppler imaging assists the identification of the origin of the cavernosal arteries and allows for accurate angle correction from the colour Doppler signal yielding a true velocity value on duplex imaging. Because the vessels can be more readily imaged an increased amount of data can be obtained and the changes in the arterial waveform easily monitored as the erection develops.

TECHNIQUE

1 Scan the flaccid penis; attempts should be made to pick up the cavernosal arteries and identify any areas of fibrosis or Peyronie's disease.
2 Inject the papaverine.
3 Scan the cavernosal arteries at the base of the penis bilaterally every 4 minutes for 16 minutes:

Document:

1 Maximal inflow velocity (Qmax)
2 Time to Qmax
3 Lowest end diastolic velocity (EDV)
4 delta T (dT): time to peak systolic velocity within a cycle
5 Erectile grade
6 Diameter of the cavernosal artery

Immediately following injection there is a reduction in resistance leading to increased velocity of flow in both systole and diastole seen on analysis of the spectral waveform. As intracorporeal pressure rises, the flow in diastole decreases and is usually retrograde at full erection in the normal subject (Fig. 15.3a). A 75% increase in the diameter of the cavernosal arteries demonstrates good vessel compliance.

Criteria for the diagnosis of arterial disease where there is failure to achieve a grade 3 erectile response are any of the following:

1 Qmax < 35 cm/sec at the origin of the cavernosal artery (Fig. 15.3b)
2 A difference between left and right cavernosal arteries of > 12 cm/sec
3 A dT value of > 0.1 sec
4 An absent or nearly absent cavernosal artery on colour Doppler imaging
5 A local stenosis demonstrated on colour Doppler imaging and confirmed by a sharp velocity gradient on duplex imaging
6 An abnormal collateral flow

Venous leakage should not be assessed by colour Doppler imaging if the arterial inflow is inadequate (< 35 cm/sec).

Criteria for the diagnosis of venous leakage are:

1 A sustained end diastolic velocity of > 7 cm/sec for at least 5 min of the study (Fig. 15.3c).
2 A failure to achieve a grade 3 erection

Cavernosometry and cavernosography

Cavernosometry is the measurement of pressure changes within the corpora. This may be in response to vasoactive agents or to perfusion with an isotonic

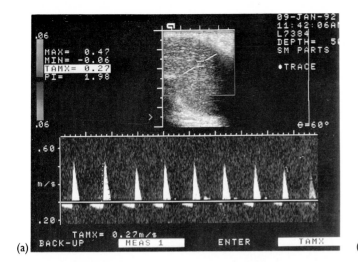

(a)

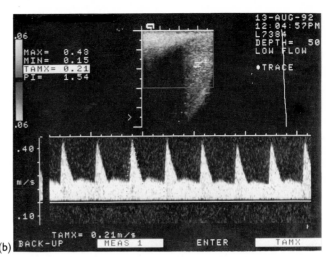

(b)

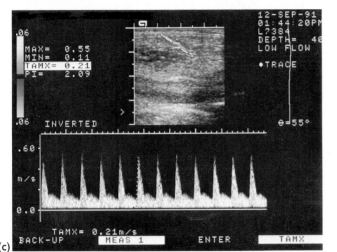

(c)

Fig. 15.3 Colour Doppler imaged arterial waveforms.
(a) Normal image showing retrograde flow in diastole. (b) venous leakage with persistent high flow in diastole. (c) arterial insufficiency with prolonged dT and poor peak velocity.

solution. Maximal information is obtained if the two are combined. Two 21G butterfly needles are required. One is connected to a three-way tap and used for papaverine injection and pressure monitoring. The other is placed in the contralateral corpora and used for infusion. The pressure transducer needed will depend on availability but all urodynamic departments will have appropriate equipment (Fig. 15.4) and most modern computerized physiological measurement systems include a programme for cavernosometry.

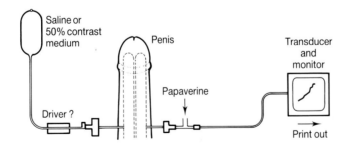

Fig. 15.4 Schematic representation of the equipment used for cavernosometry and cavernosography.

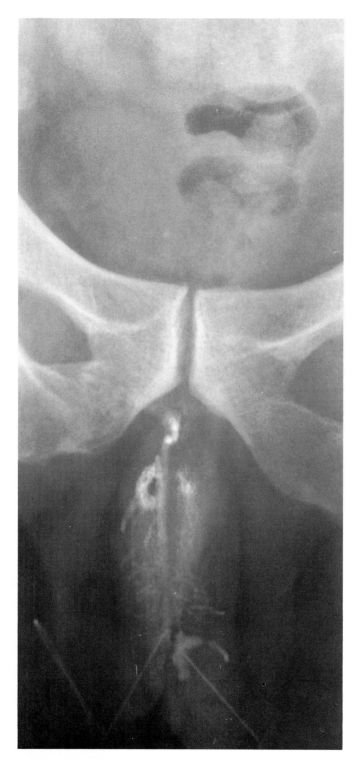

Fig. 15.5 Confirmation that both needles are correctly positioned within the corpus cavernosa prior to cavernosometry.
Contrast medium is seen outlining the sinusoids.

TECHNIQUE

1 Place both needles in the corpora and confirm their correct positions by injecting a small amount of contrast medium under fluoroscopic control (Fig. 15.5). One needle is connected to a pressure transducer via a suitable length of sterile tubing and flushed with saline, ensuring that there are no air bubbles within the transducer, tubing or needle which would dampen any changes in pressure. The pressure within the flaccid corpora is considered to be zero and so registered on measuring equipment.

2 Inject papaverine through the other needle (10 mg papaverine per decade) and monitor pressure rise in corpora over 15 min. If a grade 3 erection is obtained and the pressure rises to more than 80 mm Hg the investigation can be terminated.

3 Connect one needle to the perfusion pump and perfuse the corpora with normal saline at 40 ml/min for 5 min increasing the rate of infusion in 40ml increments until a grade 3 erection is obtained (the induction flow) (Fig. 15.6).

4 Determine the rate of infusion necessary to maintain an erection (the maintenance flow).

5 Discontinue the infusion and monitor the pressure fall in the corpora over a 2 min period.

6 If a venous leak is implied the saline infusion is replaced with contrast medium (e.g. Omnipaque 240) and spot films taken to demonstrate the venous anatomy (Fig. 15.7a and b). It is important that the intracorporeal pressure is maintained above 100 mm Hg during the cavernosography.

Document

1 Erectile grade
2 Maximum intracorporeal pressure rise following papaverine injection (DP)

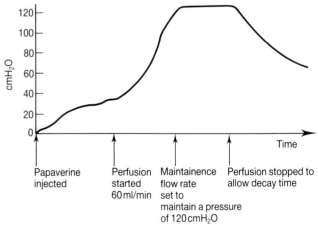

Figure 15.6 Pressure changes during pharmacocauernosography.

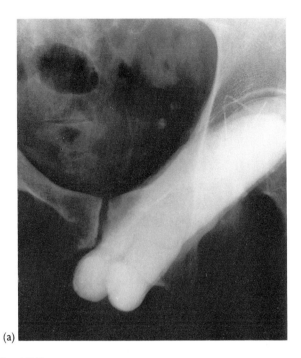

(a)

Fig. 15.7 Cavernosograms showing (a) normal response and (b) gross venous leakage in a patient with concomitant Peyronie's disease (arrow).

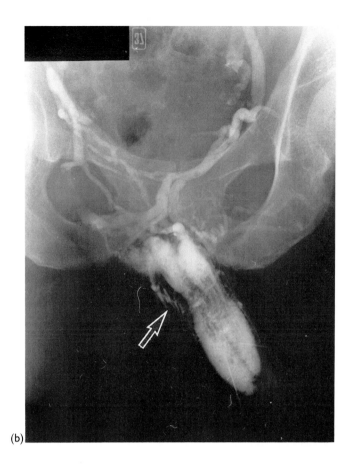

(b)

3 Induction flow (IF)
4 The maintenance flow (MF)
5 The absolute and relative pressure fall in the first 30 sec following cessation of perfusion
6 Make sure hard copy is obtained of any venous leakage

Criteria for the diagnosis of venous leakage are:

1 Erectile grade < 3
2 DP < 50 mm Hg
3 IF > 80 ml/min
4 MF > 20 ml/min
5 Intracorporeal pressure fall > 50% in 30 sec

Penile arteriography

Penile arteriography is indicated in patients for whom revascularization has a reasonable chance of success. In reality this is a small cohort of patients, mostly young men with a history of pelvic trauma or with congenital vascular abnormalities. Selective internal pudendal angiography is preferred to non-selective angiography because of the detail with which it can visualize the sites of vascular occlusion.

Bilateral 5 Fr catheters (Cook; HNB5.0–35–80–P–NS–C2) are inserted via the femoral arteries using the Seldinger technique. Before selective penile angiography, aortography is undertaken to ensure that the distal aorta, common iliac, internal iliac and proximal internal pudendal arteries are patent. The catheters are then manipulated into the internal pudendal arteries and angiography performed in the flaccid state. A vasoactive agent is then administered either intracavernosally or directly via the catheter and further selective angiograms performed (Fig. 15.8a and b). After the procedure the femoral puncture sites must be observed for haematoma formation.

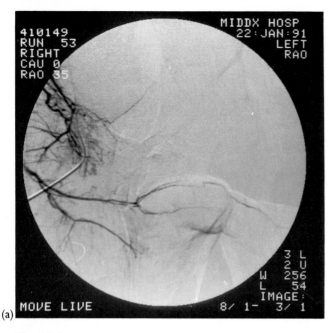
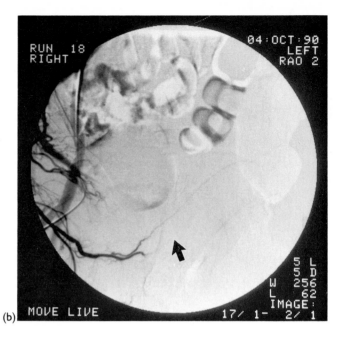

Fig. 15.8 Selective penile arteriograms showing (a) normal study and (b) occlusion of the cavernosal artery (arrow).

Complications

All these investigations are potentially frightening for the patients and are usually uncomfortable at best. In some, the adrenergic drive that results will prevent full smooth muscle relaxation from occurring within the penis. This is an important cause of false positive results and the observer should try and note if patient apprehension is compromising the interpretation of the test. Any measure which reduces anxiety levels should be taken, thus behind closed doors is better than behind closed curtains.

At the end of the procedure, firm pressure is applied to the penis after removal of the needles for a minimum of 2 min. Haematoma formation is a recognized complication.

Priapism can be expected in 4% of patients and, if not treated early, the risk of significant long term damage is increased. Appropriate instructions regarding action if the induced erection lasts longer than 2 h or is painful must be given to the patient. Priapism is treated by aspiration and if this fails to induce detumescence an intracorporeal injection of a vasoconstrictive agent (metaraminol or noradrenaline) is used. Alternatively, Aramine, 1 mg, can be injected into the corpora and repeated at 5–10 min intervals, monitoring the systolic blood pressure and doubling the dose of each injection until a total maximum of 10 mg is given. In extreme cases surgery may be required.

SUGGESTED FURTHER READING

KRANE RJ, GOLDSTEIN I, de TEJADA IS. (1989) Medical progress, impotence. *New England Journal of Medicine* **321**: 1648–59.

KRYSEWICZ S, MELLINGER BC (1989) The role of imaging in the diagnostic evaluation of impotence. *American Journal of Radiology* **153**: 1133–39.

LUE TF, TANAGHO EA (1987) Physiology of erection and pharmacological management of impotence. *Journal of Urology* **137**: 829–36.

MUELLER SC, WALLENBERG-PACHALY H, VOGES GE, SCHILD HH (1990) Comparison of selective internal iliac pharmacoangiography, penile brachial index and duplex sonography with pulsed Doppler analysis for the evaluation of vasculogenic (arteriogenic) impotence. *Journal of Urology* **143**: 928–32.

QUAM JP, KING BF, JAMES EM *et al* (1989) Duplex and color Doppler sonographic evaluation of vasculogenic impotence. *American Journal of Radiology* **153**: 1141–47.

WESPES E, DECLOUR C, STRUYVEN J *et al* (1986) Pharmaco-cavernometry-cavernography in the diagnosis of impotence. *British Journal of Urology* **58**: 429–33.

CHAPTER 16

Prostate Biopsy: techniques and applications

Matthew D. Rifkin

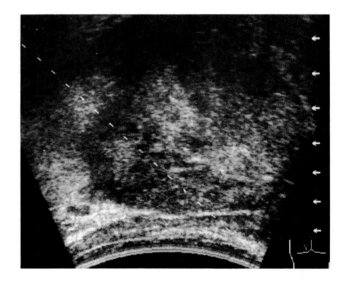

INTRODUCTION

Prostate cancer is the most common malignancy in the world. It is also the most frequently diagnosed and the second most lethal cancer in the American male population. Its prevalence and clinical significance is similar in most of the western world. The American Cancer Society estimates that over 130000 new cases will be diagnosed each year in the USA alone and over 32000 men will die from the disease in North America. Additionally, these numbers have been increasing at an alarming rate over the past 30 years.

The ability to diagnose prostate cancer has not been specific by any of a variety of clinical parameters. For example, while the suspicion of prostate cancer is raised by an abnormal digital rectal examination (DRE), the diagnosis is not specific. Cancer can be suspected by an elevation of the serum prostate-specific antigen (PSA) level. However, no levels are pathognomonic for cancer. A number of benign processes can also elevate the PSA value. An abnormality on the endo (trans) rectal ultrasound (US) may also raise the suspicion of an abnormality of the gland which may potentially be malignant. However, this study is also not diagnostic for a specific disease process. Some benign processes such as calculi, cysts, postinflammatory change, fibrosis, atrophy, unusual cases of benign prostatic hyperplasia (BPH) may mimic or suggest the presence of cancer. The determination of the presence of malignancy requires tissue.

A number of techniques can be used to acquire tissue. It can be obtained from a transurethral resection of the prostate (TURP) (performed because of the presence of benign prostatic disease and clinical symptomatology) or a transurethral biopsy of the prostate (performed during cystoscopy). However, specifying the site from which the tissue is retrieved is not possible with these techniques. Percutaneous biopsy of the prostate is the only technique which is able to obtain tissue from a specific area within the gland.

Conventional digital biopsy guidance has, until the advent of ultrasound, been the main approach for prostate biopsies. This approach can position the needle using either a transperineal or transrectal approach. However, while the palpating finger may delineate a nodule, the ability to position a biopsy needle dirictly into a specific area may not always be possible. Imaging guidance is needed to position a needle accurately into a specified region or mass.

However, imaging guidance, other than by ultra-sound is difficult. Computed tomography cannot identify intrinsic pathology within the gland. Thus, it is not possible to place the needle within a suspicious area. While magnetic resonance imaging (MRI) can identify as many focal lesions as ultrasound, because of the size of the magnet bore, and subsequent difficult access, MRI is not useful as a guiding tool. Ultrasound-guided biopsy is the only accurate and simple technique (with or without imaging) to obtain tissue consistently from a specific suspicious area.

INDICATIONS FOR PROSTATE BIOPSY

There are a number of clinical reasons for which it may be necessary to obtain tissue from the prostate.

Palpable lesions
Abnormal serum markers
Follow-up after treatment for prostate cancer

Table 16.1 *Indications for prostate biopsy*

A palpable lesion found during a digital rectal examination

There are a number of benign processes which can mimic cancer on DRE. Some of these may be tissue specific by ultrasound but many are not. The sonographic findings of some cancers (Fig. 16.1 and 16.2) may mimic the ultrasound findings of certain benign processes, such as focal inflammation, atrophy and others. In these cases, biopsy may still be needed. Other processes, i.e. calculi, cysts and others, can mimic carcinoma on DRE. However, biopsy may not be indicated if the ultrasound findings are specific.

Abnormal serum markers

If the PSA level is not normal or the prostatic acid phosphatase level is above normal, prostate cancer may be suspected. In these cases, because of the suspicion of possible cancer, even if a palpable abnormality is not present, biopsy may be indicated.

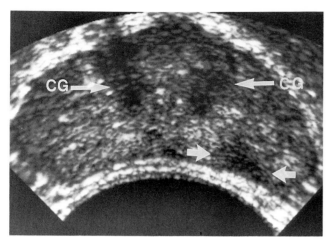

Fig. 16.1 Axially oriented endorectal sonogram demonstrates a hypoechoic area (arrows) involving the posterior aspect of the left side of the peripheral prostate. The periprostatic fat is intact. CG = central or inner gland benign prostate hyperplasia (BPH).

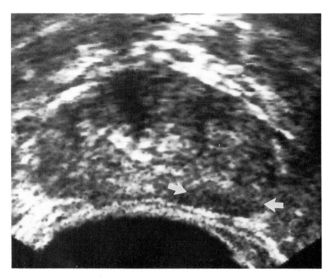

Fig. 16.2 Axially oriented endorectal ultrasound demonstrates a hypoechoic mass (arrows) involving the left posterior aspect of the prostate.

Follow-up for treatment of a known prostatic carcinoma

A patient with prostate cancer who has been treated with a non-surgical approach, i.e. radiation, hormonal or chemotherapy, may need to be assessed for regression or progression of tumour. Following the initial treatment, repeat biopsies may be indicated to evaluate any possible residual or recurrent cancer.

CONTRADINDICATIONS FOR PROSTATE BIOPSY

Prostate biopsy is a simple procedure and there are relatively few contraindications for the procedure.

1 The most significant are patients with bleeding diatheses. Because it is difficult to occlude bleeding vessels, within the prostate after biopsy, it can be difficult to stop bleeding that may occur in these patients.
2 Other contraindications include patients who are taking blood-thinning agents. While patients on coumadin or other strong anticoagulants should cease their medication prior to biopsy, it has even been suggested that aspirin ingestion may also be a relative contraindication to performing a biopsy. However, biopsies have been performed on men on low-dose aspirin without complication, so clinical decisions on each individual must be made about whether cessation of medication may be necessary.

APPROACHES TO BIOPSY

There are a number of approaches to biopsy. The major two being core biopsy and aspiration cytology.

Core biopsy

A variety of needles (i.e. Tru-Cut, Vim-Silverman or another type), when used appropriately, obtain a core or a large piece of tissue. This is useful for both diagnosing a specific disease process and, in cases of prostatic cancer, it also permits accurate histological grading of the malignancy. Both may also be useful when planning treatment. The risk of complications increases when the larger sized needles are used, although there is not a significant increase in the rate of complications between a 18 and 22 gauge needles. However, the larger 14 gauge needles (i.e. the Tru-Cut and Vim-Silverman needles), do represent a potentially significant increased risk than the smaller 18–22 gauge cutting needles. The smaller needles usually yield diagnostically adequate specimens, and they have almost totally replaced the larger needles, regardless of the technique of biopsy employed.

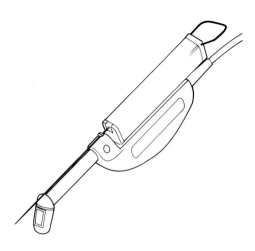

Fig. 16.3 Automatic trigger device loaded into an oblique 'end-fire' transrectal ultrasound probe for endorectal biopsy.

The introduction of the automatic trigger devices or 'guns' using 18 or 20 gauge cutting needles has revolutionized the percutaneous approach to prostate biopsy in the past few years (Fig. 16.3). The devices permit a more 'rapid' biopsy to be performed than with conventional cutting needles. In appearance and in use, the needles utilized with the automatic trigger devices are similar to conventional biopsy needles. These needles can be used 'free hand' or coupled to a mechanical triggering device or 'gun' that ensures rapid, safe extraction of a core of tissue. The use of these devices with slightly smaller gauge needles has increased the speed of biopsy, decreased the discomfort and significantly decreased the rate and risk of complications (i.e. bleeding and/or haematoma) without loss of diagnostic accuracy.

Aspiration cytology

Fine-needle aspiration has been used extensively in Europe and for prostate biopsy it is now becoming more frequently used in the USA. The aspiration cytology needle is smaller than a core biopsy needle, usually 22–23 gauge, and thus the risk of complications is reduced. While diagnostic accuracy of aspiration is, in experienced hands, comparable to the large-core biopsy, its diagnostic accuracy is very dependent upon the individual experience of the cytopathologist. Diagnosis is made by the microscopic analysis of a few groups of cells or even a single abnormal cell. Because of the small number of cells being evaluated, histological grading of cancer is often not possible.

COMPARISON OF DIGITAL TO ULTRASOUND-GUIDED BIOPSIES

The conventional digitally guided biopsy (both for the transperineal and the transrectal approaches) is performed with a finger in the rectum to assist in accurate needle placement. With the finger palpating the area of abnormality, the biopsy needle is guided toward the lesion through the perineum or rectal wall into the lesion. Either of these approaches can be performed with both the core biopsy and aspiration cytology techniques.

The digitally guided biopsy of a palpable mass is not perfect. While only about 50% of palpable areas of the prostate are malignant when biopsied using conventional digitally guided biopsies not all negative biopsies are truly negative. It has also been estimated that the false negative rate for these palpable lesions is only approximately 10%. However, the actual percentage is significantly higher. Studies have shown that the false negative rate of digitally guided biopsy may be closer to 40%.

ULTRASOUND GUIDED BIOPSY PATIENT PREPARATION

Depending upon the US approach, biopsy is performed in either the lithotomy or lateral decubitus position. The transperineal approach, no longer utilized as often as it has been in the past, usually requires the patient be positioned in the lithotomy position. The transrectal biopsy can be performed with the patient in the decubitus position. Ultrasound-guided biopsies utilizing small gauge needles or automatic 'trigger' devices do not usually require local or general anaesthesia or sedation. Thus, biopsies may be performed in an outpatient setting.

Prior to biopsy, one must ensure that the patient

does not have a significant bleeding disorder, bruise easily or is currently using anticoagulation. Some physicians feel that use of salicylates is a contra-indication and patients should abstain for 10 days prior to biopsy; others feel that chronic or periodic use of low-dose salicylates is not a contraindication.

Evaluation of patients with a 'battery' of haematologic studies, i.e. prothrombin time (PT), partial thromboplastin time (PTT), platelet count etc. is usually not required if all clinical parameters are normal. Antibiotics should be given prophylactically prior to transrectal biopsies to minimize the risk of sepsis.

Transrectal biopsy

The development and production of 'end' or 'oblique end-fire' transducers has permitted the transrectal approach using ultrasound guidance, to become an easy and the most acceptable technique. Especially produced guides which can be placed into or directly over the endorectal probe and guide the biopsy needle have been made (Fig. 16.3). Each different transducer usually requires its own unique guide. A complex arrangement of preparation of the equipment is often necessary. Each device has different requirements. The transrectal biopsy tecnique has been shown to be highly successful for biopsying both large and small lesions.

The biopsy is performed as follows:

1 Prebiopsy antibiotics are given (at least 30 min) pior to biopsy. A cleansing enema is administered prior to the procedure.
2 To identify the lesion, a preliminary sonogram is performed.
3 The endorectal guidance probe is prepared with a biopsy guide.
4 The patient is placed in lateral decubitus or if necessary, lithotomy or knee–chest position.
5 The endorectal probe is placed in the rectum.
6 The probe is positioned until the lesion is re-identified and the line of sight of needle placement position is visualized on the screen (Fig. 16.4).
7 Under sonographic guidance, the needle is placed through the guide, through the rectal wall, into the lesion in the prostate (Fig. 16.5).

Either core or cytology aspiration biopsies can be performed using this technique.

A major benefit of the transrectal approach is minimal patient discomfort: no anaesthesia is needed. The one potential significant problem of the technique is the risk of sepsis (reported in up to 2% of all patient biopsies). Reported results also show that the rates of other complications are increased compared to the transperineal approach. For example, the incidence of haematuria may be as high as 37% of cases, the incidence of blood in the bowel movement about 10% and the incidence of haematospermia may reach 5%. However, the clinical significance of these 'minor' complications does not appear to be increased.

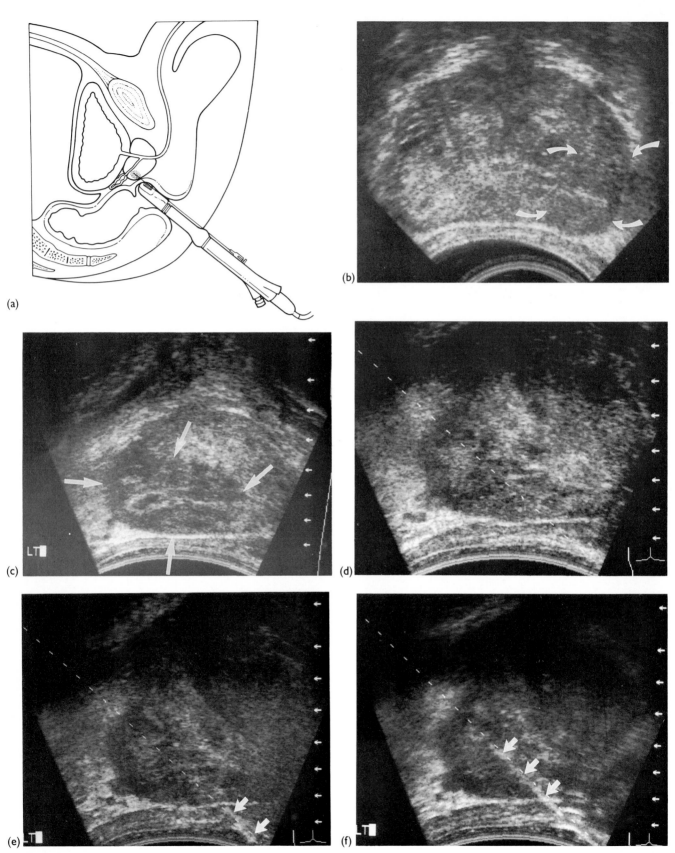

Fig. 16.4 (a) The theoretical approach to a transrectal biopsy is shown in the line diagram. (b) The lesion (arrows) is identified on the axial scan and (c) the 'end' or 'oblique angled' longitudinal image. (d) The line of sight of the biopsy (dashes) is placed so that the needle would traverse directly through the lesion. The needle during biopsy (arrows) is seen as it traverses into (e) the rectal wall, and into (f) the lesion.

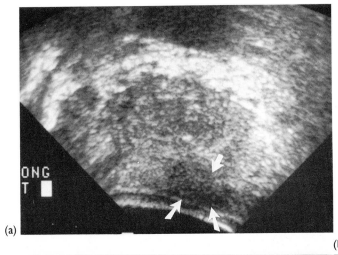

(a)

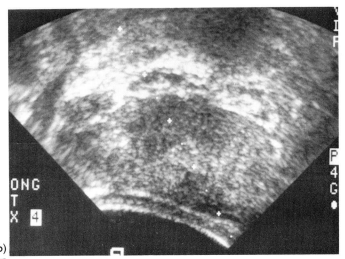

(b)

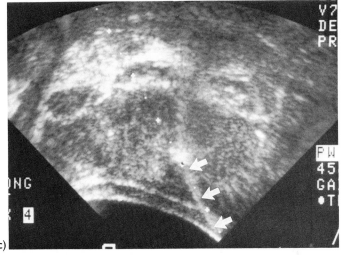

(c)

Fig. 16.5 (a) Longitudinal scan demonstrates lesion (arrows). (b) The line of needle placement is positioned over the lesion. (c) The needle (arrows) is identified in the lesion during biopsy.

TRANSPERINEAL BIOPSY

Initially, ultrasound presented images in a sagittal orientation. These required a perineal biopsy approach. This approach has been replaced in most instances by the transrectal biopsy technique. Yet, there will be times the transperineal route may be needed to perform this biopsy.

When performing an endorectal ultrasound-guided biopsy, the biopsy needle can be guided into the prostate in two fashions: (1) 'free hand' guidance without direct attachment of the needle to the endorectal probe, or (2) with the use of a biopsy guide that is attached or 'fixed' to the probe. The latter technique is useful because it simplifies the procedure. A variety of attachments is available, depending upon the specific equipment utilized. Generally, each manufacturer supplies their own guide and procedure for its use.

When performing the transperineal approach, the patient is usually placed in the lithotomy position. In general, the biopsy can be performed as follows (Figs.16.6 and 16.7):

1 An initial diagnostic endorectal sonogram identifies a lesion
2 The probe is removed
3 Prebiopsy precautions are observed
4 The patient is placed in the lithotomy position
5 Since the procedure is performed in a sterile fashion, antiseptic solution (i.e. Betadine) is applied to the perineal area. Since no faecal material will contaminate the biopsy site and a sterile approach is used, no cleansing enema or antibiotics are usually needed. However, if a patient is unusually prone to develop infection, i.e. has cardiovascular disease, mechanical prosthesis or other prosthetic devices implanted, or other risks, then prophylactic antibiotics should be given.
6 Local anaesthesia (1% xylocaine) is applied to the skin and subcutaneous tissues with a 25 gauge

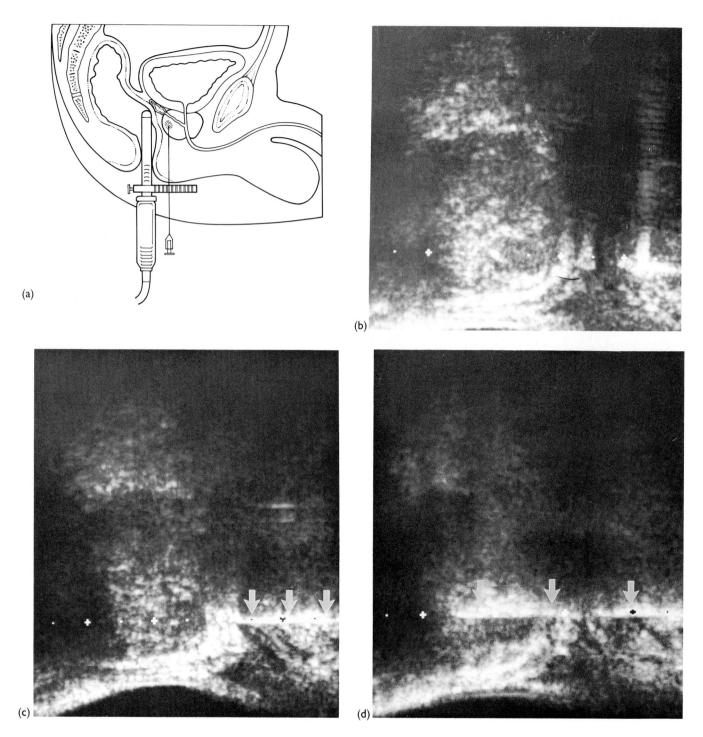

Fig. 16.6 (a) The theoretical approach of the transperineal biopsy with a 'fixed' guide attached is shown in the line diagram. (b) Using a longitudinally oriented side fire transducer, the line for needle placement (dots and crosses) is placed so that the needle will traverse directly through the lesion. The reverberation artifacts as the needle is placed into the soft tissues are also seen. (c, d) The needle (arrows) is seen as it progressively traverses into and through the prostate capsule and then directly into the lesion during biopsy.

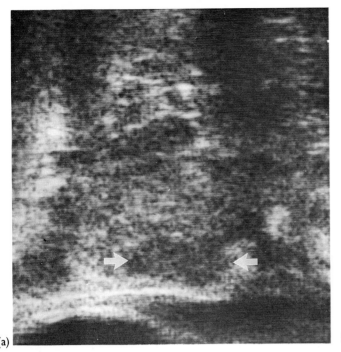 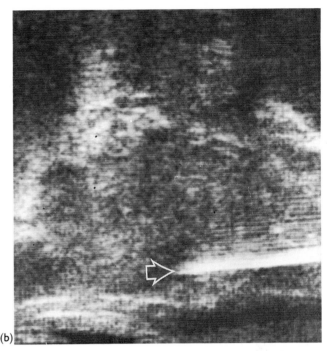

(a)　　　　　　　　　　　　　　　　　　　　　　　(b)

Fig. 16.7 (a) Longitudinal scan shows lesion (arrows). (b) The needle (arrowhead) can be angled if necessary during biopsy.

needle to the area of needle insertion, i.e. to the right, or left or in the middle.

7　The probe with guide attached is replaced into the rectum. The one hand holding the probe is no longer sterile. The other hand, which remains sterile, holds the needle. The needle should be identified at all times when in the ultrasound image's field of view.

8　The probe is rotated clockwise or counterclockwise to re-identify the lesion and is then 'fixed' in that position.

9　A 22 gauge spinal needle is placed through the guide (or if the 'free hand' technique is used, along the probe's parallel axis) into the already anaesthetized subcutaneous tissues. Anaesthesia is then given to the deeper soft tissues and the prostatic capsule area.

10　With the lesion identified advance the needle through the guide and into the prostate. (For 'freehand' biopsies, the needle is placed into the perineum parallel to the crystals on the longitudinally oriented probe.)

11　If an aspiration cytology biopsy is to be performed, a thin gauge needle is placed into the most caudad area of the lesion. A 10–20 ml syringe is tightly attached and suction is applied. The needle is carefully and gently moved in an 'in–out' fashion and simultaneously rotated slightly in a 'clockwise–counterclockwise' fashion without releasing suction. When the aspira-

tion is completed, the suction should be released very gently, and the needle removed. The material is expressed immediately onto a slide and smears made or the material can be expelled into an appropriate solution (consultation with the pathologist to ascertain the appropriate material is essential).

12　If a core biopsy is being performed, the needle should be placed just caudad to the lesion (as described in step 11). Under conventional sonographic guidance, the biopsy is performed. The material obtained by biopsy should be 'fixed' in formalin or other preservative.

The sagittal orientation allows identification of the exact site of tissue extraction so that even small areas of sonographic abnormality can be clearly identified and biopsied. Both large and small gauge needles can be clearly and consistently identified. The use of a biplane probe or 'end fire' permits rapid sweeping back and forth to identify the lesion and confirm the position of the biopsy needle in both planes.

POSTBIOPSY PROCEDURES

Following the biopsy a number of precautions should be followed:

1 If a patient has undergone a transrectal biopsy, broad–spectrum antibiotics should be given for 2–5 days following the procedure.
2 The patient should not be discharged unless a urine specimen is clear, or if haematuria has occurred, has started to clear.
3 The patient should be instructed to drink fluids freely and extensively.
4 The patient should be educated regarding the risks and symptoms of (uro) sepsis.

Transrectal approach	Transperineal approach
No anaesthesia required	Local anaesthesia required; minimal patient discomfort may be experienced
Accurate biopsy	Accurate biopsy
Multiple sites can be biopsied at one sitting	Requires more anaesthesia to biopsy multiple sites

Table 16.2 *Comparison of the benefits of transrectal versus transperineal sonographic-guided biopsy*

	Incidence (%) of complications in the transrectal approach	Incidence (%) of complications in the transperineal approach
Haematuria	37	2
Blood in bowel movement	9.4	0
Blood in ejaculate	5.0	0
Sepsis	2.0	0
Vasovagal reaction	Complication not reported	1

Table 16.3 *Comparison of complications of transrectal and transperineal sonographic-guided biopsy*

COMPARISON OF THE TRANSRECTAL WITH THE TRANSPERINEAL APPROACH

Both the transperineal and the transrectal approach to endorectal sonographically guided biopsy of the prostate are equally accurate. However, there are differences (Table 16.2), for example:

1 Complications (Table 16.3). The transrectal approach appears to have a significantly higher incidence of haematuria, haematochezia, haematospermia and sepsis. The transperineal approach has a minimally increased risk for a vasovagal reaction. Except for sepsis, these are usually not clinically significant complications. Sepsis is the most significant complication, and its frequency appears to be proportional to the size of the needle employed; that is, the larger the biopsy needle used, the higher the risk of sepsis. When using the transrectal approach, it has been estimated that up to 85% of patients will have positive blood cultures following biopsy.
2 Patient positioning. The transperineal approach is usually simpler to perform in the lithotomy position. The transrectal biopsy can be performed in either the lithotomy or the decubitus position.
3 Accuracy. Both techniques are equally accurate in obtaining tissue from a specific area.

Needle tract seeding along the site of biopsy with implantation of of malignant cells has been estimated to be a rare occurrence in prostate biopsy although, theoretically, it can occur.

CONCLUSIONS

Sonographically guided biopsy is not always necessary in order to biopsy palpable lesions. However, when a palpable mass is biopsied by conventional means, repeat biopsy with ultrasound guidance may be indicated. Also, subtly or nonpalpable lesions may have to be biopsied with endorectal sonographic control.

The type of biopsy is, in general, a matter of preference. Both the transperineal and transrectal approaches appear to be equally accurate. Although the number of complications increases with the transrectal approach, these may not be clinically significant. The approach used should be according to the individual's preference.

SUGGESTED FURTHER READING

Burkholder GV, Kaufman JJ (1966) Local implantation of carcinoma of the prostate with percutaneous needle biopsy. *Journal of Urology* **95**: 801–4.

Catalona WJ, Scott WW (1986) Carcinoma of the prostate. In: *Campbell's Urology*, 5th edition, pp. 1463–534. Edited by Walsh PC, Gittes RF, Perlmutter AD, Stamey TA. WB Saunders, Philadelphia.

Grayhack JT, Bockrath JM (1981) Diagnosis of carcinoma of prostate. *Urology* **17**(Suppl): 54–60.

Lee F, McLeary RD (1987) Ultrasound guided biopsy techniques: transperineal and transrectal. Presented at the Second International Symposium on Transrectal Ultrasound in the Diagnosis and Management of Prostate Cancer, Detroit, Michigan, 21–22 September.

Rifkin MD (1988) *Ultrasound of the Prostate*. Raven Press, New York.

Rifkin MD, Alexander AA, Pisarchick J, Matteucci T (1991) Palpable masses in the prostate: superior accuracy of US-guided biopsy compared with accuracy of digitally guided biopsy. *Radiology* **179**: 41–2.

Rifkin MD, Choi H (1988) Endorectal prostate ultrasound: implications of the small peripheral lesions in hypechoic endorectal US of the prostate. *Radiology* **106**: 619–22.

Rifkin MD, Dahnert W, Kurtz AB (1990) State of the art: endorectal sonography of the prostate gland. *American Journal of Radiology* **154**: 691–700.

CHAPTER 17

Urogenital prostheses

Simon A. V. Holmes, Timothy J. Christmas and Roger S. Kirby

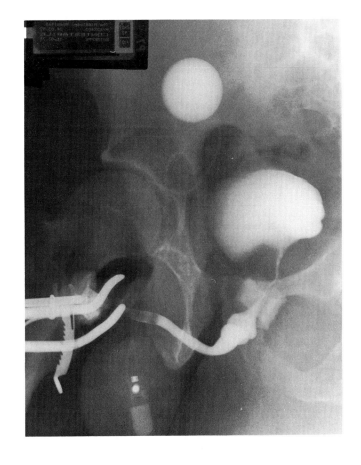

UROGENITAL PROSTHESES

Through the last two decades the use of implantable prostheses in all surgical specialties has grown exponentially, and urology is no exception. There are now a number of different urogenital devices which can be implanted within the urinary tract or genital organs. These prostheses may serve roles of cosmetic enhancement or the functional replacement of diseased or damaged urogenital components.

PENILE PROSTHESES

The first materials used as prostheses for achieving penile rigidity were sections of rib implanted into the dorsal aspect of the penis to create an os penis. The first use of silicon, as a single rod prosthesis was described in 1966, but it was not until 1973 that the twin penile prosthesis that we would recognise today was first used. There are now a number of design variations with an estimated 17000 being inserted annually in the USA. They are now all paired devices which occupy the whole of each corpus cavernosum and are either simple rigid or semi-rigid rods, giving the penis a degree of permanent rigidity (Fig. 17.1a and b), or have an hydraulic component that allows inflation of the prosthesis. The simple nonhydraulic rods are cheaper and are associated with a lower incidence of complications. They may be rigid, hinged to allow downward positioning of the prosthesis or malleable along the whole length for variable positioning. The inflatable rods are expensive, may develop mechanical failure and have a separate hydraulic device, usually in the scrotum, for inflation.

The success of implantation of these devices is dependent on patient selection. Penile prostheses enable the patient to have sexual intercourse but do not restore normal erections, improve libido or restore ejaculation and patients should be made aware of this. The prostheses can be inserted under general or spinal anaesthesia through a variety of different incisions. Hospital stay is 1–3 days although day case insertion may soon be possible. Insertion is simple, adopting a few basic principles: parenteral broad spectrum antibiotics, local antiseptics, accurate measurement of corporal length and suitable selection of device.

The complications that can occur from insertion are related to either mechanical failure of the device or the anatomical sequelae of implantation such as infection, erosion, migration (Fig 17.2) and pain. Mechanical failure of the rod prostheses is rare but fracture can occur. Inflatable prostheses are more mechanically complex and consequently susceptible to leakage, tubal disruption, cylinder rupture and reservoir malfunction. The hydraulic fluid contains contrast medium and so plain radiography of the lower abdomen and pelvis can diagnose the malfunction in most cases. Radiology is also used to identify the prosthesis after migration, with implants being found in the upper thigh, and hydraulic reservoirs have been known to migrate into the peritoneal cavity. Erosion of the prosthesis, due to ill-fitting or infection, can lead to perforation of the corpora with or without urethral involvement. Prosthesis infection is the most common complication, occurring in about 2% of all cases (1.8% with rods, 2.6% with inflatable prostheses). *Staphylococcus epidermidis* is the commonest infecting organism and the next commonest are the Gram negative gut organisms. If

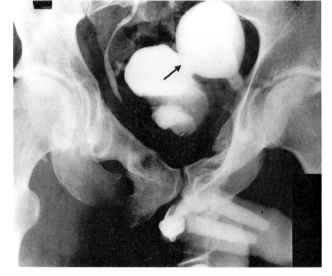

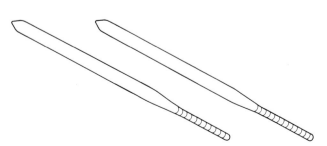

Fig. 17.1 (a) Semirigid penile prostheses which give the penis a permanent degree of semirigidity. (b) Penile rods have been implanted into this patient with impotence following pelvic fracture. A Brantley Scott artificial urinary sphincter has also been inserted to control continence. The reservoir (arrow) is adjacent to the bladder on this excretory urogram.

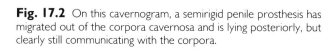

Fig. 17.2 On this cavernogram, a semirigid penile prosthesis has migrated out of the corpora cavernosa and is lying posteriorly, but clearly still communicating with the corpora.

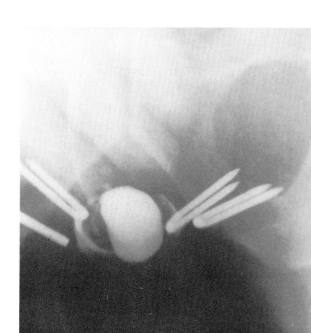

Fig. 17.3 The Kaufmann device.
An expandable prosthesis is stapled to the inferior pubic rami. By injecting contrast medium into the device and enlarging it, passive resistance to the posterior urethra is achieved. Should the device deflate, it can be refilled with contrast medium under fluoroscopic control.

infection is suspected early surgical intervention is indicated with removal of the device and irrigation of the cavity with antiseptics before fistulae or corporeal fibrosis occur.

THE ARTIFICIAL URINARY SPHINCTER

The first proposed use of an artificial device to act as a urethral sphincter was by Foley in 1947. The device at that time was impractical but superficially resembled the prostheses we now have available, involving an inflatable cuff mechanism. The first devices to be used clinically, such as the Kaufman device (Fig. 17.3), were passive compression devices that maintained continence by obstructing the bulbar urethra with voiding achieved by elevation of the intraabdominal and intravesical pressures. This nonphysiological mechanism of action was responsible for the high failure rate of these devices. The first implantable artificial urinary sphincter (AUS) with an inflatable cuff to see clinical use was described in 1973 by Scott. The AUS was constructed of silicon-elastomer and had a complex system of pumps, valves and reservoirs to inflate and deflate the cuff, which wrapped around the urethra. The fluid within the system was usually contrast medium so that an assessment could be made of the possible cause of their relatively frequent mechanical failures. Current devices contain an isotonic solution of contrast medium (10% Hypaque) unless precluded by patient allergy. A number of subsequent modifications were made to this device over the next 10 years, improving the reliability and efficacy with each development, culminating in the AS–800 which is now the most widely used model (Fig. 17.4). It consists of a single pressure regulating balloon reservoir and a separate pump unit which contains a deactivation button which when depressed will release the cuff during voiding. A further model, currently being developed, will have the reservoir and pump in one unit and will also have a subcutaneous chamber that can be injected percutaneously to alter the volume and hence the pressure within the cuff mechanism.

The AUS is suitable for a wide variety of problems resulting in incontinence in both adults and children including congenital and acquired causes of

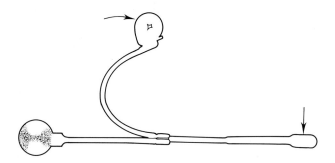

Fig. 17.4 The Brantley Scott artificial urinary sphincter. The cuff (curved) can be deflated by squeezing the control mechanism mounted in the scrotum or labia (arrow).

Radical prostatectomy	36%
TURP*	30%
Myelomeningocoele	15%
Stress incontinence	5%
Neurogenic	5%
Pelvic trauma/surgery	4%
Other	5%

*TURP = transurethral resection of the prostate gland.

Table 17.1 *Approximate causes of artificial sphincter use in the USA*

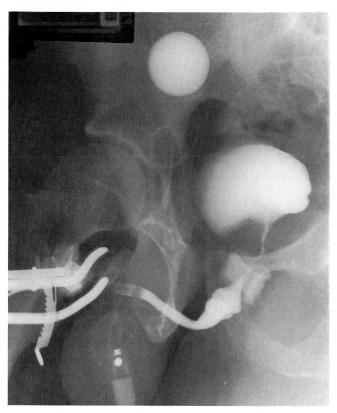

Fig. 17.5 Ascending urethrogram in a patient with a Brantley Scott prosthesis.
The intracuff urethra is attenuated (arrow). The pump (open arrow) is within the scrotum.

the neuropathic bladder, female incontinence and postsurgical causes. A review of the aetiologies is given in Table 17.1. The best results are obtained in those patients with normal bladder function who simply have a weak sphincter. Bladder hyperreflexia, sphincter dyssynergia or diminished bladder compliance are associated with poorer results, and these should be identified in the pre-operative investigations. Prior to surgery scrupulous antisepsis is essential combined with prophylactic broad spectrum antibiotic administration. The cuff, which comes in a variety of sizes, can be placed around the bladder neck or the bulbar urethra, with the bulbar urethra preferred in men and the bladder neck in women unless previous trauma or surgery renders the tissue unsuitable. The balloon is sited in the prevesical space and the pump mechanism is placed immediately below the skin in the scrotum or labia majora. Postoperatively the bladder is drained with a urethral catheter for 1–3 days and the pump mechanism is checked once prior to hospital discharge. Use of the AUS can begin after teaching the patient the technique about 4 weeks after insertion.

The complications of AUS insertion are in principal similar to penile prostheses. The commonest, failure of the cuff to close, is caused by either pressure atrophy of the tissue beneath the cuff or a leak in the device. Other problems include a kink in the tubing and debris in the system. Leakage and kinking can usually be demonstrated by plain radiography as can loss of fluid volume in the system if there are postoperative films available for comparison. The cuff is the commonest site for leakage to occur followed by the balloon. Cuff efficiency can be more accurately assessed by urodynamic investigation if necessary (Fig. 17.5). Infection of the device is a serious problem and inevitably leads to its removal. Infection most commonly presents as a cuff erosion which should be suspected by pain on manipulation or burning in the perineum. Confirmation of the diagnosis should be performed by cystoscopy and not urethrography as this investigation may contaminate a sterile erosion and usually fails to demonstrate a small one. Plain X-ray may show the presence of gas forming around the device. Despite all prophylactic measures infection can still occur in up to 10% of implanted devices.

TESTICULAR PROSTHESES

The loss or lack of a testis in a male has been shown to be as psychologically traumatic as the absence of a breast or uterus to a woman. This appears to be irrespective of age and thus prostheses should be considered in most cases of testicular loss. Since the first reported testicular prosthesis in 1941 a number of materials have been used including vitallium, glass, lucite, Gelfoam, Dacron and polyethylene until the silicon-gel filled silicon rubber prosthesis was introduced in 1973 (Fig. 17.6). These have a natural consistency, the correct weight and come in four different sizes. Prosthetic insertion in children therefore requires replacement with a larger one as the child grows. The commonest indication for insertion is the undescended or atrophic testis, followed by testicular tumours and torsion. Prostheses should be inserted via the inguinal route and can be done so at the time of original exploration or at a second procedure if there is any risk of infection.

The main complication of testicular prostheses is infection which can be followed by wound dehiscence and prosthesis extrusion. This occurs in about 5% of operations and most commonly occurs with insertion after epididymo-orchitis. Other complications include pain, scrotal contraction and, rarely, rupture of the silicon envelope.

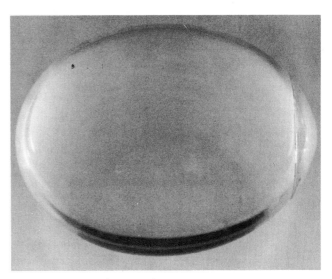

Fig. 17.6 Testicular prosthesis.

of some prosthetic materials with particular reference to the risk of malignant transformation. A number of devices have been withdrawn from the market and national licensing bodies are demanding stringent confirmation of their safety. There have, however, been no reports of these problems in urogenital devices and the risks would appear to be very small. The overall use of urogenital prostheses continues to grow and if more biocompatible materials are found many more devices will become available.

SUMMARY

The most serious complication that occurs with prostheses is infection. Bacteria have been shown to adhere readily to the surfaces of implanted materials where they exist within a biofilm. This is a glycocalyx layer produced by the micro-organisms which protect the bacteria within, making them resistant to the effects of antibiotic treatment. Thus infection of a prosthesis is almost inevitably followed by prompt removal of the device, as the infection can not be eradicated. The infection may then be followed by loss of function of the affected organ and replacement of the prosthetic device is either prohibited or at least made more complex. Migration and mechanical failure of the devices is another common problem and radiologists may be asked to locate the prostheses or identify the source of trouble within their mechanics. Attention has recently focussed on the long-term biocompatability

SUGGESTED FURTHER READING

BRANTLEY SCOTT F (1989) The artificial urinary sphincter. *Urological Clinics of North America* **16**: 105–17.
LATTIMER JK, VAKILI BF, SMITH AM *et al* (1973) A natural feeling testicular prosthesis. *Journal of Urology* **110**: 81–3.
PETROU SP, BARRETT DM (1990) The use of penile prostheses in erectile dysfunction. *Seminars in Urology* **8**: 138–52.

Index